SEX POSITION FOR COUPLES:

KAMA SUTRA ADVANCED GUIDE FOR A BETTER SEX, MAKE YOUR SEXUAL LIFE EXPLOSIVE

ALEXIA WINNIS

TABLE OF CONTENTS

INTRODUCTION

Believe it or not, it's not primarily a sex manual.

Kamasutra of Kamasutra is an ancient book about sex education. This book is often mistaken as the book of Tantric Sex. In fact, it is like a discourse in the importance of sex in human life. It narrates various facets of corporeal acts done by men and women. It is a book of educating us bout deep intimacy and the relationship between two genders, male and female.

The Kama Sutra, believed to be written during the second or third century C.E. by the Hindu Vedic philosopher Vatsyayana, is a guide to virtuous living, filled with aphorisms on the nature of love and the importance of family life. It tells of finding a life partner and creating a harmonious relationship, navigating the challenges of extramarital relationships, balancing family and duty and the need to make a living - as well as a variety of positions for sexual intercourse.

"Sutra" in Sanskrit means treatise; "Kama" refers to desire, pleasure or sex. Thus: Treatise on Desire/Pleasure/ Sex. For Vatsyayana, however, desire/pleasure/sex holds a different meaning than for us world-weary moderns overly familiar with commoditized sex. Desire, pleasure, and sex in the Kama Sutra are contextualized, seen as part of a worldview in which men and women dance together in the arts of love and families and larger networks of relations.

Since Burton's day, the Kama Sutra has come to be used as a shorthand way of referring to exotic eroticism. The sections of the book which describe sexual positions have come to stand for the whole book, with numerous books (and movies) published that picture photogenic models enacting these positions for our edification. As it turns out, even ancient texts can be broken down and used in simplistic ways to feed the modern yearning for sexual wholeness. But we moderns have it backward: sexual wholeness does not come via abstracting the "good parts" of a wise guide to life that happens to have the patina of age. Vatsyayana's work locates this grounded sexuality in the context of loving and respectful relationships with clear boundaries.

WHAT IS KAMA SUTRA?

Did you know the Kama Sutra was written by a celibate scholar? Or that the Kama Sutra revolves around a man's pleasure? Or that only about 20% of the book is about sexual positioning? Interestingly, most people know about Kama Sutra and yet they don't know what it is about.

After being with the same partner for several years, many couples are desperately curious about how to spice up their sex life. Stuck for options, they secretly tiptoe down the "sex" section of the bookstore to get a peek at the Kama Sutra nudie pictures and acrobatic sexual positions. Titillated, they buy the book only to have it sit untouched and lonesome in their nightstand drawer forevermore.

Unfortunately, they failed to understand that Kama Sutra is not a sex-quick-fix; rather, it's a comprehensive way of looking at their sexuality. As such, it has remained under its mystical Eastern shroud since it first hit pop-culture in the early 1980s. Truthfully, the Kama Sutra isn't all that complicated and it's a great way for couples to keep their sex fun and fresh over the long term.

So what is Kama Sutra? It was meant as a pillow book. Whereas our Western culture believed in not talking about sex and leaving kids ignorant until their wedding day, Eastern culture had the opposite viewpoint. When a young person became engaged, they were given a "pillow book", which was their technical guide on how to have sex. Vatsyayana happened to create the world's most famous pillow book.

Tradition believes Vatsyayana was a celibate scholar who lived sometime around 4th century AD. He did not write the Kama Sutra per se; rather, he was a compiler and editor of all the information that existed during the very rich Gupta period. Interestingly, Vatsyayana believed that sex itself was not wrong, but doing it frivolously was sinful.

Therefore, "Kama" literally means desire and "Sutra" signifies a thread or a thread of discourses. While most of us believe the Kama Sutra is all about sexual positions, 80% of the book gives insights on how to make love a divine union, how to act like a responsible citizen, how to handle your household, etc. It's a discourse or a marriage manual to troubleshoot all the sticky points a young man or young woman will face in their pending marriage. Brilliant. And then there are the infamous 64 positions which have launched hundreds (maybe thousands) of books, videos, and websites. Vatsyayana believed there were eight ways to make love, multiplied by eight positions. A veritable smorgasbord.

What many people don't realize is that the Kama Sutra's focus is to give the man the maximum amount of sexual pleasure. Eastern culture believed that, for the man to get the maximum amount of gratification, he first had to bring the woman to full arousal. Why? The more sexual energy she had, the more likely her energy would cross over to give him a bigger, better orgasm.

What does that translate to? Our quickly-becomes-boring Western get-on, get-in, get-off type of sex cannot begin to rival Kama Sutra's sex because it is about the entire sexual experience. Kama Sutra's sex has a beginning, middle, and end-instead of just focusing on the middle as Westerns do. First, the Kama Sutra gives instructions on how to prepare yourself and your environment for lovemaking. It then talks about multiple ways to have foreplay to "energize" the woman (yeah!). It then shows many different options for positions. The possible combinations are endless, enabling you to mix-up sex every time.

You may be asking, "If Kama Sutra is so great, why aren't more people jumping on the bandwagon?" Well, if you go authentic and read Richard Burton's original translated version of Vatsyayana's work, it is deathly boring. Did I mention complicated? He talks about yonis and bulls and other euphemisms that are unfamiliar to our Western sensibilities. It's intimidating and off-putting for the average couple. Luckily, Anne Hooper came out with Kama Sutra for 21st Century Lovers. It's the best version I've seen on the store shelf because it is written in understandable language and the photos are superb. Or if you want to go more authentic, Deepak Chopra is trying to cash in on his name with his beautiful version of Kama Sutra.

If you've done the math, yes Kama Sutra takes more bedroom work. Time starved couples look at it, roll their eyes and say, "No thanks." Please remember though, good sex gives you and your relationship a much-needed injection of energy. The ten or fifteen minutes of extra time will take your sex from blah to bravo.

A BRIEF LOOK AT THE KAMA SUTRA

The ancient Sanskrit text of the Kamasutra, more commonly known in western culture as the Kama Sutra, was originally written by Mallanaga Vatsyayana and is believed to be a masterwork on the ways of Love in all its forms. The Kama Sutra is just one, though the most notable, of a larger collection of ancient Indian texts known as the Kama Shastra or Discipline of Kama. These texts were original of a religious nature and common theology holds that the collection was handed down to mankind by Shiva's doorkeeper, Nandi the sacred bull, after hearing the god, Shiva and Parvati, his wife having relations. The session so inspired the sacred bull to make utterance which was later recorded and passed down to mankind for their benefit. It is believed that the present form of the Kama Sutra is a compendium that was gathered at some point in the second century CE.

Etymologically speaking, Kama Sutra can be broken down into two Sanskrit words; the first being Kama, which is a reference to the Hindu god of Love, using the same name. In common language, it conveyed the ideas of desire, wish, intention, pleasure, and love, especially in a sexual connotation. In chapter two of Richard Burton's translation of the text, Kama is translated as "the enjoyment of appropriate objects by the five senses of hearing, feeling, seeing, tasting and smelling, assisted by the mind together with the soul. The ingredient in this is a peculiar contact between the organ of sense and its object, and the consciousness of pleasure which arises from that contact is called the Kama."

The second word, Sutra refers to a discourse delivered on a set of concise rules. Thus Sutra has the connotation of a technical study or manual. Thus, the Sutra was intended to educate the reader in the field of its particular study.

Taken together, the words Kama Sutra imply a

technical text on the aspects of properly enjoying the stimulation of the five senses and the demonstration of Love. Unfortunately, the simple wording of the title has led to many misconceptions regarding the text and it is to be noted that the Kama Sutra is neither a sex manual or a sacred religious text, though it does incorporate both aspects into its writing. While the text is explicit in details of a sexual nature and also intones highly religious themes, it was intended to put the Kama into context with the other two aims of ancient Hindu life, Dharma and Artha. This is evidenced by Vatsyayana's opening discussion of these three aims at the beginning of the text.

These three terms are described as relating to Virtue (Dharma), Material Prosperity (Artha) and Pleasure (Kama) and they were to be pursued in that order. The first *q*uality almost always took precedence over the secondary when two of these pursuits were at odds, though there were a few exceptions to this rule. Thus being virtuous was to be sought more than wealth but pleasure would fall secondary to the pursuit of material gain in the Hindu way of life. The Kama Sutra was intended as a guide to show how to properly achieve all three goals and their proper places to achieve Moksha, the liberation from the cycle of reincarnation.

THE SECRETS BEHIND THE KAMA SUTRA

Now when we think about The Kama Sutra, we tend to think of a book entailed several different sexual positions used to enhance overall sexual pleasure, but is all there is to it?

A Guide To Relationships And Life

The Kama Sutra was designed in India many centuries ago and contains information not only about sexual enhancements but about relationships, marriage, and life. Western civilization first became enthralled by its complexity mainly in the area of sexual intercourse and as a result, proceeded to extend upon the information in this area.

Nowadays we see a lot of information claiming to be relevant to the Kama Sutra, however, the majority of readings out there contain very little information related to this ancient script. When we think of The Kama Sutra we have to try and understand the reasoning behind it.

Why It Was Designed

The Kama Sutra was designed as a means of bringing two people together in an arranged marriage to increase the emotional level of the relationship. This would then cause fewer complications in other areas of life and a peaceful marriage could then be ascertained.

There are a lot of texts out there that contain information not just about sexual positions and the like, but also about increasing the amount of love you and your partner can share in your relationship. These are the readings that you should try and stick too.

Sexual Positions Of The Kama Sutra

Now people are incredibly attracted to the variety of sexual positions inside The Kama Sutra, and why not? They are a great way to increase the amount of pleasure not just in the bed, but also reflecting in everyday life. A little extra excitement in the bedroom can do wonders for personal self-esteem!

There are many types of positions that The Kama Sutra conforms to such as - Anjou Style, The Twining of a Creeper, The embrace of the thighs, The embrace of the breasts and many more. It's pointless trying to describe each one of these positions individually so if you plan to try a couple out, it's probably best to by one of the many books out there on sexual positions of The Kama Sutra.

Try to remember one thing when it comes to this small piece of The Kama Sutra - what level of emotional commitment do you and your partner share? The physical nature of sexual intercourse can only take you so far in terms of the amount of pleasure you will receive. A strong emotional attachment can create an unbelievable sense of euphoria that I promise you won't see coming!

KAMA SUTRA - THE CONTENT OF THE KAMA SUTRA

The Kama Sutra written by Vatsyayana consisted of seven sections further divided into thirty-six chapters. We will discuss each of these sections to glean the details of what Vatsyayana was trying to convey in the Kama Sutra and the importance he placed on specific subjects.

•Section One - Introductory

The first section of the Kama Sutra consisted of five chapters explaining the contents of the manuscript, the three major aims, and priorities of life according to the Hindu belief system of the day, the acquisition of knowledge, suitable conduct for the well-bred townsman and various reflections on intermediaries who assist the lover in his enterprises.

•Section Two- On Sexual Union

The second section of the Kama Sutra consisted of ten chapters on the stimulation of desire, various forms of embraces, caressing and kisses, marking a partner with the use of the fingernails, biting and marking a partner using the teeth, on positions of copulation, explanations of sexual practices such as slapping with the hand and moaning that accompanied the practice, evidence of virile behavior in women, superior coitus and oral sex practices, along with preludes and conclusions to the game of love. There are 64 types of sexual acts described in this section which has become the part of the Kama Sutra for which the book is most widely known.

*Section Three - About The Acquisition Of A Wife

Section three of the Kama Sutra consists of Five chapters on the forms of marriage, how to relax and obtain the girl, how to manage alone when a suitable wife cannot be found and the union by marriage.

*Section Four- About A Wife

Section four consists of counsel to the various types of wives a Hindu gentleman may have had. Two chapters are dealing with the conduct of the wives. The section of the Kama Sutra yields advice to the solitary wife in how she should conduct herself. This section of the Kama Sutra also explained the conduct of the chief wife and other wives in a household with multiple wives and concubines.

*Section Five - About The Wives Of Other People

This section of the Kama Sutra consisted of six chapters on the behavior of women and men. It included advice on the methods of seducing another mans wife, including encounters for getting acquainted, examination of sentiments, the tasks and advantages of go-betweens, the king's pleasures such as his harem and ways the brave could circumvent security measures and enjoy those pleasures themselves, as well as the proper behavior of a Hindu gentleman in the gynoecium or women's apartments.

*Section Six - About Courtesans

Section Six of the Kama Sutra consisted of six chapters on making the best use of the advice of the assistants on choosing lovers, the search for a steady lover, the courtesans skill set and ways of making money, how best to renew friendship with a former lover, creating occasional profits and dealing with profits and losses associated with being a courtesan.

•Section Seven - On The Means Of Attracting Others To One's Self

The two chapters of section seven of the Kama Sutra deal mainly with thoughts on improving physical attractiveness to others and arousing a weakened or failing sexual power.

THE IDEOLOGY OF THE KAMA SUTRA

When we think of the Kama Sutra, we automatically start to think of different sexual positions, commonly seen in books on tantra, but is that all this ancient script is about or is there more than meets the eye with this commonly mistaken text?

A Whole Relationship Guide

Now The Kama Sutra was not just designed as a guide to better sex, but as a way to bring two people together closer than ever before. The ideology behind The Kama Sutra, best describes some of the modern teachings about how to increase the amount of love and connection between you and your partner.

The teachings of sexual intercourse comprise just a small fraction of the teachings in The Kama Sutra. It was first written as a way to bring two people from an arranged marriage together so they could connect, mainly to make life easier for the rest of the family.

The Pleasurable Side Of The Kama Sutra

Now I'm not going to stand here and say that sex is not a big part of the Kama Sutra, because it is and several of the techniques have been used very successfully to increase the level of love and connections in relationships. So what are some of the best positions to put into practice?

The Embrace Of The Thighs

Sounds kinda kinky, doesn't it? This is where one of the lovers pushes hard on one or both of the thighs of the lover between his or her thighs. Of course, you may have already come across this position before in the bedroom. This particular position is one of four 'embracing' positions outlined in the Kama Sutra and is used to create a tighter grasp around the woman's vagina.

Lying Down Kama Sutra Positions

Another group of positions in The Kama Sutra is the lying down positions, which include: the widely opened position, the yawning position and the position of the wife of Indrani. The first position requires the female to arch her back and lower her head. The second requires the woman to raise her thighs and the third is when the woman places her thighs with her legs doubled on them upon her sides.

Of course, this is just a fraction of the number of sexual positions outlined in The Kama Sutra and it would take many years to perfect them all, so you better get started!

MALE AND FEMALE ENHANCEMENT OF THE KAMA SUTRA

Vatsyayana freely admitted that even the god of love can sometimes have a poor aim. When he does, strange unions form as can be understood by the following quote from the Kama Sutra: "Sometimes Kama, absent-minded, throws his arrow haphazardly. Thus one sees strange couples assembling. A man and a woman who should not have been brought together. They attract criticism, mockery and yet, 'badly-matched' love defies time! This hare-man, thin and graceful, adores his elephant wife, as powerful as a giant.

Their tastes, their preoccupations, their bodies, are discordant. But they adore each other! And, in the games of love, their harmony is perfect. The hare-man knows all the subtle caresses that arouse his wife. Making use of Apadravyas, he increases the size of his frail lingam. There are all kinds of them in the pleasure room: gold armband, precious wood tube, ivory bracelet. They choose them according to how their lovemaking progresses."

We have all met couples that just don't appear to be well suited for each other and yet they seem to thrive on the other company. Just as the couple mentioned in the Kama Sutra, we find very thin men with much larger women or small-statured ladies in love with men who appear to be mountains. It isn't a new fad by any means. What advice did the Kama Sutra offer these couples to make their sexual encounters more pleasurable for both parties?

Ancient Male Enhancement Secrets Of The Kama Sutra

Aside from the above recommendation of supplying a less than adequate lover with attachments to increase length and girth, the Kama Sutra offered another bit of advice. This came in the form of a recipe for an ancient form of male enhancement. Let's take a look at this ancient secret in the words of the Kama Sutra itself.

"First rub your lingam with wasp stings and massage it with sweet oil. When it swells, let it dangle for ten nights through a hole in your bed, going to sleep each night on your stomach.

After this period use a cool ointment to remove the pain and swelling. By this method men of insatiable sexual appetite, manage to keep their lingam enlarged throughout their lives."

That prescription makes those Apradavya's, or sexual accessories mentioned above, look like a walk in the park. I don't know about you, but, I would rather be laughed at by every woman I ever met than try that particular cure.

Ointments For Female Enhancement From The Kama Sutra

It seems that while Vatsyayana's advice may have been a bit masochistic for the men, he was a little easier on the ladies. In the Kama Sutra, he described two different ointments for different purposes.

For the ladies who were of a size that was a bit too large for their man to accommodate them, the Kama Sutra provided the following insights: "By applying an ointment made from crushed Barleria leaves to her yoni, the elephant woman can spend at least one night discovering the delights of being a doe."

If she happened to overdo the effector was just too small to accommodate a larger male, to begin with, he had a different ointment. He went on to say, "Likewise the doe can use honey mixed with powdered roots of Lotus, Madder, Sal (tree of aromatic gum), the Blue Lotus and the Mongoose plant to accommodate a stallion for one night."

STANDING POSITIONS OF THE KAMA SUTRA

The Kama Sutra of Vatsyayana is world-renowned for its wisdom and incite that can be found in its writings. It is particularity well know for a very brief passage that discusses a variety of sexual positions and aids in the lovemaking process. In this article, we will discuss three of the numerous standing sexual positions of the Kama Sutra.

What Were Vatsyayana's Thoughts On The Kama Sutra Standing Positions?

To quote the author, "There are some lovers who despise soft beds and cozy cushions. Their pleasure is heightened by danger or discomfort. Some choose places where their union may be discovered; others practice the most hazardous positions. Others still seek risk and difficulty. Their pleasure room is a garden where they lay open to being seen." With those words in mind, let's consider three of the standing positions mentioned in the Kama Sutra.

•Knee - Elbow

A position rendered much simpler and safer with the assistance of a support structure such as a wall, the Knee-Elbow is a very erotic position for lovers to experiment with. In the words of the Kama Sutra, "If you lift your lover bypassing your elbows under her knees and gripping her buttocks while she hangs fearfully from your neck, it is Janukurpara," which translates to the Knee Elbow. This is a very interesting position with a lot of possibilities for the athletic among us though, if you are a bit out of shape, you might consider a strict exercise and training regimen before this experience.

•Stag

The stag is a leaning position of the Kama Sutra that provides for a very sensual experience for both partners. The Stag position is accomplished by the woman standing with her back to her partner, usually assisted by leaning against a steady structure such as a wall or fence. The man approaches from behind her and joins with her. Then both can make whatever motions suit their own needs and the needs of their partner. Another variation puts the woman standing but then leaning forward at the waist to brace herself with her hands by touching the ground.

•Tripod

"If you catch one of her knees firmly in your hand and stand to make love with her while her hands explore and caress your body, it is Tripadam (the Tripod)." - The Kama Sutra

Aptly named, the Tripod of the Kama Sutra is yet another position for the contortionists among us. With this position, only three out of the pairs four feet will touch the ground at any given time. In the different variations, the woman will wrap one leg around her partners waist and rest her heel on the back of his knee, rest her foot on her partners chest just above the heart, stretch one leg up and over her partners shoulder or have her partner extends his arm and cup her foot in his hand while they are making love.

A Word Of Caution

While these three positions may sound enticing, please be sure to know your physical limits before beginning. As awkward as these positions can be to get in and out of, it can be even more awkward to explain to your in-laws or coworkers just how you pulled your hamstring or slipped a disc in your back.

GROWING CLOSER WITH THE EMBRACING POSITIONS OF THE KAMA SUTRA

The Kama Sutra of Vatsyayana was intended as a lesson in proper decorum and relationships between Hindu couples of its time. Just as their modern counterparts, ancient couples sought after a deeper level of intimacy with each other and a feeling of closeness. It penned the Kama Sutra in hopes of helping his peers to achieve the goals of life, including the goal of Sutra, and to put these goals in a proper perspective. One of the recommended forms in the Kama Sutra was the positions of Embracing as they provided for special closeness.

Why Is Embracing Important?

It is quite amazing how much feeling can be communicated by an embrace or hug. As children, we are comforted in times of pain or sickness by mothers loving arms. As we grow older, we still seek out that close bond with others as a way to feel loved and appreciated. With an embrace, we can express condolence, affection, protection or comfort. In the Kama Sutra, Vatsyayana recognized the importance that an embrace could hold in a relationship between lovers. He realized that the simple act of embracing could convey the deep emotions and security that the mates provided for each other and a feeling of connecting their souls. With these thoughts in mind, he recommended the Embracing positions of the Kama Sutra.

What Are The Embracing Positions Of The Kama Sutra?

Vatsyayana related a variety of embracing positions in the Kama Sutra with two varieties for standing embrace being the The Twining of the Creeper which the Kama Sutra describes as, "When a woman, clinging to a man as a creeper twines round a tree, bends his head down to hers with the desire of kissing him and slightly makes the sound of sut sut, embraces him, and looks lovingly towards him." and the Climbing of a Tree which they explained as being, "When a woman, having placed one of her feet on the foot of her lover, and the other on one of his thighs, passes one of her arms around his back, and the other on his shoulders, makes slightly the sounds of singing and cooing, and wishes, as it were, to climb up him in order to have a kiss."

The Kama Sutra goes on to relate several embracing positions to be applied at the time of sexual union. These were known as The Mixture of Sesamum Seed with Rice and The Mixture of Milk and Water. Both of these positions were intended to induce closeness and a sense of melting two bodies into one.

Vatsyayana's Kama Sutra went on to describe four lesser embraces as well that involved more specific areas of the body rather than the complete embraces mentioned above. These four embraces are conveyed to us as The Embrace of the Thighs, The Embrace of the Jaghana (or. the part of the body from the navel downwards to the thighs), The Embrace of the Breasts and The Embrace of the Forehead.

ALL THE GOALS OF THE KAMA SUTRA

The Kama Sutra was written by Mallanaga Vatsyayana in ancient Sanskrit. It was written by the purusharthas of Indian tradition as its basis. These purusharthas are commonly referred to as the four main goals of life. By ancient Hindu tradition, these goals were key to escaping the cycle of reincarnation or being reborn in different castes and states according to the actions of a previous lifetime. These goals were Dharma, Artha, Kama, and Moksha. The first three goals, Dharma, Artha, and the Kama are portions of everyday existence whereas Moksha was the highest goal achieved by reaching the three earthly goals. The achievement of the goal, Moksha, meant that one would be released from the cycle of death and rebirth.

According to Vatsyayana, as translated by Sir Richard Francis Burton, "Dharma is better than Artha, and Artha is better than the Kama. But Artha should always be first practiced by the king for the livelihood of men is to be obtained from it only. Again, the Kama being the occupation of public women, they should prefer it to the other two, and these are exceptions to the general rule." (Kama Sutra 1.2.14) Thus it can be seen that each of the goals was ranked according to its value in the scheme of things.

•Dharma - Virtuous Living

The first goal is Dharma or Virtuous Living. This goal implied leading a life of moral values and doing good works. The individual seeking to achieve Dharma would seek to avoid ill will and injury to others. In some traditions, the pursuit of Dharma was even extended to animal and insect life to the point that a man was not allowed to kill an insect. While many people would not consider the Kama Sutra to be a particularly moral text, there is a very high placement given to Dharma or Virtuous Living. Dharma is considered such a high goal that whenever two motives conflict, Dharma is always the path to be followed.

•Artha - Material Prosperity

The second goal of life, according to Vatsyayana and his Kama Sutra, was the pursuit of Artha or Material Prosperity. This goal made certain that a man's household was well provided for. As long as a man's living did not interfere with his Virtue, it was considered to be a distinguishing point to be gainfully employed. The proper Hindu gentleman worked very hard to make certain that the goal of Artha was satisfied by making a good life for him and his household.

•Kama - Aesthetic And Erotic Pleasure

Kama or Aesthetic and Erotic Pleasure is the third goal of life according to the Kama Sutra. This goal also lends its name to the title of the text as Vatsyayana peened the ancient Sanskrit tome as a guide to putting the pursuit of Kama in its proper place. The Kama is the lowest of the three motives and was considered "the occupation of public women" or prostitutes. The Kama was the pursuit of physical pleasure and had its proper place in the life of a Hindu gentleman. This motive has become the focal point for many individuals in their definition of the Kama Sutra even though the goal of the text was to put Karma in its proper place as the lowest of the three motives.

For those looking for spiritual enlightenment along the Hindu path to Moksha or for those who seek a simple way of putting life into perspective, Vatsyayana's Kama Sutra has much to offer in the way of teaching.

THE MORAL REPERCUSSIONS OF THE KAMA SUTRA

At the time Vatsyayana penned the words of the Kama Sutra, he had no idea what he was beginning. He and his contemporaries were highly educated, religious men of the Hindu faith. The work that Vatsyayana put onto parchment was not intended as a corrupting influence but was more the advice of one who had traveled a path and wanted to share the knowledge of the journey. Even though, Vatsyayana refers to "public women" or prostitutes, explaining the differences between them and their uses, and coaches his male students on the proper way to seduce a married woman while admitting that relations with another mans mate are to be avoided, he was a fairly moral man for the society of his time. If he and his contemporaries could see the later works of today, they might question our moral fiber.

What Did Vatsyayana Start?

Vatsyayana published the Kama Sutra as a way of sharing his knowledge but to some societies, this knowledge would seem ill-gained. He spoke of the use of consorts, both male and female, and of various forms of sexual intercourse. These positions came as quite a shock to Victorian-era English men and women when Sir Richard Burton published the first English translation of the work. While it outwardly brought fainting, shuddering and a conflagration, in private people were titillated by the work and it began to eat at the back of their minds just how some of those positions worked and whether that male enhancement recipe that called for the stings of a wasp did work permanently. Burton, himself having three Indian mistresses, was quoted to say, "We British never knew of this kind of love-making. Had we known, we would not have ruined the lives of so many British virgins." This comment was made after his visit to a prostitute of the day. While folks claimed an aversion to the subject matter, they were privately drawn to it and the morals of the society began a subtle change.

As the secrets of the Kama Sutra slowly leaked out, the common man thought to himself that this or that new idea sounded *q*uite interesting. For some time when the missionary position was the only church-sanctioned union, some of the ideas of the Kama Sutra must have sounded very intriguing. Now and then a recipient of the Kama Sutra's knowledge would decide to give something a try and come back with a sore back or a pulled tendon but with each torn ligament there was also a tear in the morals of the society.

How Far Did This Influence Reach?

The influence of the Kama Sutra did not stop with the English countryside. Far from it, the influence has spread to nearly all parts of the world and has become even more pervasive as the *q*uality of communication has increased. With the Internet and the eased restrictions on the publications of printed material, the Kama Sutra finds a larger following all the time. Unfortunately, many people have forgotten Vatsyayna's original goal for the Kama Sutra which was to put sex and its pleasures in their proper perspective. Society has become very promiscuous and *q*uick to go for what feels good to the individual. Thus we find a moral breakdown unparalleled by any other time in history.

SECRET KAMA SUTRA SEXUAL POSITIONS

Kama Sutra has become incredibly popular in the past few years. Many people are taking to this ancient text as a way of improving the amount of excitement in the bedroom. Many sexual positions are talked about in The Kama Sutra, but only a certain few seem to create enormous amounts of pleasure.

•The Dog

The dog was designed as a way of increasing pleasure by the man being behind the woman in a position that is unbelievably more pleasurable for the woman than for the man.

It has become one of the most used Kama Sutra positions in the world due to its ease of use. It has become common practice for sexual partners to use this position more often than any other. If you are planning on trying something new and you haven't tried the dog, then you and your partner are in for a treat.

•The Lotus

The lotus is described as when the man is sitting cross-legged with the woman on top. This again is certainly a very popular position and was designed in one of the first Kama Sutra's back many centuries ago. Most people like to switch from this position into another. There are many positions to go to from The Lotus, including; the right angle(the man standing with the woman laying on her back), the clip(man lies down and the woman leans back on her knees) and many others.

I'm sure that you have done the lotus on numerous encounters, which you probably don't remember as it is a position that most people switch in between during intercourse.

•The Visitor

The Visitor is probably the most intimate of sexual positions outlined in The Kama Sutra. It is when both the man and woman are standing and in the past, you have likely been in this position before. Because the two of you are standing, most of the eroticism is taken out of the mood and replaced with a feeling of total connection.

If you and your partner are deeply in love, the visitor can magnify that love tenfold. Worth giving a go next time.

The Kama Sutra was firstly designed not as a guide to sex, but as a guide to total relationship building. Most people tend to forget this and focus more on the physical side of this ancient text. One of the main teachings in the Kama Sutra discusses how pleasure can only be maximized in the bedroom if you and your partner share a strong sense of connection. Focus on your relationship and it will reflect in the bedroom.

THE PROPER APPLICATION OF
THE KAMA SUTRA

When Vatsyayana first penned the Kama Sutra, he had a few important things in mind. He wanted to teach proper Hindu gentlemen of his time the lessons about the major goals in life and how these goals were to be obtained. One of those goals was Sutra, or pleasure derived from experiences. Though the term Sutra could mean pleasure from other than erotic or sexual stimulus, the Kama Sutra has come to be synonymous with sexually learned and those who have studied it find themselves sought after as sexual partners.

While the sexual aspect of the Kama Sutra alone is very educational, the further development of attached emotions and philosophy was also important to Vatsyayana when he wrote the text. This is evidenced by the following quotation from Vatsyayana's Kama Sutra - "Such passionate actions and amorous gesticulations or movements, which arise on the spur of the moment, and during sexual intercourse, cannot be defined, and are as irregular as dreams. A horse having once attained the fifth degree of motion goes on with blind speed, regardless of pits, ditches, and posts in his way; and in the same manner a loving pair become blind with passion in the heat of congress, and go on with great impetuosity, paying not the least regard to excess. For this reason, one who is well acquainted with the science of love (Kama Sutra), and knowing his strength, as also the tenderness, impetuosity, and strength of the young women, should act accordingly. The various modes of enjoyment are not for all times or all persons, but they should only be used at the proper time, and in the proper countries and places."

What Was Vatsyayana Trying To Say?

Vatsyayana knew that people were very interested in the study of human sexual behaviors. After all, mankind has not existed for so many years without some first-hand knowledge of the subject. However, as an avid scholar of human behavior, he also knew that knowledge of the art of making love was not, in itself, enough to provide for happy relationships. Physical attraction can only reach so far and two people who cannot communicate will not remain together for very long. He also knew that there is a time for everything. There are occasions where certain displays would be unwelcome or even inappropriate.

Throughout the majority of Vatsyayana's text, he tried to show readers of the Kama Sutra how important the emotions and feelings that accompanied congress were. He advised repeatedly to have an understanding of one's mate and their needs and personality. Without such knowledge and understanding, a relationship would be doomed to failure and unhappiness.

How Does It Apply Today?

Despite advancement and civilization, the human creature is much the same as it was eons ago. We still share the same emotions of our ancestors through our choice of the display may differ. What Vatsyayana wrote in the Kama Sutra of his time is still very poignant today. For a relationship to work, more than physical action is required. One must apply themselves to learning their partner's quirks and needs. Listen to your partner and act on what you have heard. As Vatsyayana understood so well, Love is made with the heart, not with the body. Share emotions with your partner and the sexual relationship will benefit also.

KAMA SUTRA OIL

It's a cold, snowy evening. The wind howls outside and whips around the house like a wild beast trying to gain entry to the home. Inside, the house is warm and dry. Soft music is playing in the background. There is a roaring fire in the fireplace, which is providing the only light in the room, with a blanket spread out on the floor before it. You and your partner lay on the blanket sipping a finely chilled glass of champagne and feeding each other chocolate-covered strawberries. You have been reading the Kama Sutra and have been utilizing the wisdom of Vatsyayana to restore the fires of passion. In so doing, you have discovered the value of touch and massage as a way of providing intimacy with your partner. Just this afternoon, you stopped at a shop in the next town and bought a selection of massage oils, the Kama Sutra Oils of Love. It is going to be a very enjoyable evening for both you and your partner.

What Is Kama Sutra Oil Of Love?

Kama Sutra Oil of Love is a delectable massage oil that provides for luxurious evenings of gentle relaxation and intimacy. The oils are scented and flavored to increase the pleasure and arousal of both partners by stimulating the sense of taste and smell. These flavorings and scents commonly include chocolate, raspberry, cherry almond, mint, tangerines, strawberries and vanilla creme.

In addition to the olfactory and flavorful pleasures, Kama Sutra Oil of Love also offers tactile pleasures with a warm, tingly sensation and the feel of slippery luxurious oils. These tactile pleasures offer themselves well to an erotic and sensual massage. With the skin being the largest sensory organ of the human body, with literally millions of nerve receptors, massage can be a very relaxing and intimate experience, as well as the physical rewards of reducing stress and toxins in the body.

How Do I Use Kama Sutra Oil?

To make the best use of Kama Sutra oil, it is recommended to warm the product first by soaking the bottle in a bowl of warm water. This preparation can be made while your partner takes a hot bath or shower to begin the relaxation process.

When your partner emerges from their bathing routine, make sure the room is warm enough for their comfort and have them lie face down so you can begin by massaging the back. Put a liberal amount of the warm oil in your hands and begin with short, lighter strokes and work up to heavier, long strokes. For the heavier strokes, use your body weight rather than the strength of your arms as this will greatly increase the amount of time you can spend comfortably giving a massage.

Massage involves a few basic motions that can be repeated and switched around in varying patterns for various effects. These keystrokes are:

•**The Glide** - This involves long smooth strokes using the entire hand that follows the curves of your partner's body.

•**The Palm** - For this stroke, using the palms of your hands as the pressure points fan out across the body pushing up and then lessening the pressure and returning to the starting point.

•**Push-Pull** - This is a simple stroke performed on the sides of the body using both hands, with one hand pushing up as the other comes back in a push-pull motion.

•**The Lift** - This is a kneading, lifting stroke with the fingers lifting your partner's skin.

•**All Thumbs** - This stroke is achieved by placing direct pressure on your partner's body with the palm of your hand and using only the thumbs pressed against your partner's skin and moved in a circular motion.

With these simple motions and a little initiative, Kama Sutra oil can turn a cold, winter night into a very romantic evening.

THE FACTS ABOUT THE ILLUSTRATIONS OF THE KAMA SUTRA

People have spent hours poring over them, trying to mimic intricate poses and styles. Others have had a good chuckle at how well the name of a certain act, such as the tripod or the elephant, matched the aesthetic qualities of the pictorial evidence. Many more just stared in disbelief and said: "How did they do that?"

While the illustrations may be thought-provoking or to titillate, they are not part of the original manuscripts that Vatsyayana penned. The illustrations were added at a later date by translators as a way of making the sometimes difficult wording of the Kama Sutra more readily understood by the average reader and were never intended to be part of the original manuscript, as a common myth would imply.

How did the Kama Sutra Illustrations Get There?

Centuries after Vatsyayana first put the words to the Kama Sutra into the path of history, readers were still interested in his subject matter, perhaps even more so than his contemporaries. Unfortunately for the average reader without a knowledge of the Hindu background from which Vatsyayana had written the masterpiece, some of the language and wording was exceedingly difficult to decipher even though Richard Burton had translated the text into the popular language of the Victorian era of which he lived. People were interested in the subject matter but, as with many difficult to understand subjects, people shied away from reading long, detailed passages that were hard to comprehend in favor of books that were easier to digest.

This trend continued for quite some time before someone recognized a need for a change. Proponents of the work and publishers could no longer stand to see the masterpiece shunned because it was too difficult to comprehend so an effort to make the text more readable began. The effort led the way to illustrated copies of the Kama Sutra which we find today.

Where did the Kama Sutra Illustrations Come From?

The changes in the Kama Sutra had begun. Authors were hired to rewrite the book in the modern vernacular and as publishers decided to add illustrations to the Kama Sutra, they needed to find a source for their illustrations. One such author was Madelyn Carol Dervos who began her rewriting work in 1988 and made repeated trips to India over ten years to collect artwork for her reproduction of Vatsyayana's masterpiece. Traveling all over India and looking at many amazing pieces of art, she sought out paintings that would cause her readers to see themselves in the illustrations and was very successful in this cause. These paintings, as well as others, have since been translated into the illustrations we see in today's illustrated Kama Sutra versions.

Though the so-called original Kama Sutra illustrations may not be as original as some would lead us to believe, they do not detract from the work but do tend to enhance the reader's understanding of the wording. Illustrated or not, the Kama Sutra by Vatsyanya will remain a master text on the ways of Love.

THE CASTE SYSTEM AND THE KAMA SUTRA

In every game, there are rules to follow and lovemaking in Ancient Hindu cultures had a set of rules all its own. Vatsyayana's Kama Sutra illuminates these special provisions for us so that we might gain a deeper understanding of the principles and ideals that governed the culture of his time. Ancient Indian culture divided people into a caste system with several thousand divisions but four main groupings. These individual castes had their ranks and peculiarities.

It is commonly believed that castes were decided by a person's birth because it was believed that Karma, or what you did in life, affected the cycle of reincarnation and rebirth but it has been shown that the caste system was non-hereditary in its original form. While you could interact with people of a different caste, there were special rules of conduct and the practice was generally frowned upon.

To understand how the caste system affected lovers in the ancient Hindu culture of Vatsyayana's time, let us examine the words of the Kama Sutra itself: "When the Kama is practiced by men of the four castes according to the rules of the Holy Writ with virgins of their caste, it then becomes a means of acquiring lawful progeny and good fame, and it is not also opposed to the customs of the world.

On the contrary, the practice of the Kama with women of the higher castes, and with those previously enjoyed by others, even though they are of the same caste, is prohibited. But the practice of the Kama with women of the lower castes, with women excommunicated from their caste, with public women, and with women twice married, is neither enjoined nor prohibited. The object of practicing the Kama with such women is pleasure only."

How Did The Caste System Work?

According to other ancient manuscripts of the time, these castes were divided into four main parts called Varnas. The Varna designations were the Brahmins (teachers, scholars, and priests), the Kshatriyas (kings and warriors), the Vaishyas (traders), and Shudras (agriculturists, service providers, and some artisan groups). There was also a fifth classification deemed to be outside the caste system called the Parjanya, Antyaja or Dalits.

These were considered the "Untouchables" as they were considered as being beneath society and this was usually reserved for those with communicable diseases or held occupations that carried communal health risks or severe uncleanness. This grouping would not have even figured into the Kama Sutra because of the very presence of such an individual was considered to defile a person of a higher caste. The defiled individual was then required to bathe thoroughly and purge themselves of any impurities.

When applied to the Kama Sutra, the caste system was shown as a way of determining who safe options were for partners. It provided a measure of safety from various communicable diseases between castes as people were less likely to engage in relations with a person who was below them in the caste system.

For those seeking a lifetime partner through marriages, it also provided a way of reducing contention amongst the spouses by ensuring that both families were of the same background and thus had common ground. This also served to keep lower classes from becoming wealthy by profiting from marriages to higher classes as this was most generally avoided.

THE SOCIAL RAMIFICATIONS OF THE KAMA SUTRA

When Vatsyayana first penned the text that we today know as the Kama Sutra, he could have had no idea of the economic impact he was creating. A manuscript brought to life by a man who history has all but lost has created such legal issues through the course of history as to make it one of the most highly debated and vilified texts in publication. Let's take a few moments to reflect on the social ramifications of the Kama Sutra on Victorian culture in Great Britain.

From A Publishing Standpoint

From the publisher's standpoint, the ancient Sanskrit text has been a glowing success. This is easily evidenced by the many translators who have taken upon themselves, the task of rewriting and compiling the manuscript for the masses to enjoy. The first such translator for the English language was Sir Richard F. Burton, a British explorer who spoke no less than twenty-five languages fluently. When he discovered the text upon one of his journeys of exploration through India in 1842, he became enamored by the book and decided he must translate the text into the language of his peers back in Great Britain so that they too could enjoy the material he was now so fond of. Thirty-four years later, in 1876, Sir Richard Burton had finally finished the work of translating the Kama Sutra with the assistance of his collaborator, Forster Fitzgerald Arbuthnot, since Sir Burton could not read ancient Sanskrit himself. The first published tomes were still a long way off, however.

The Kama Shastra Society

Seven years later, in 1883, the first English copies of the Kama Sutra were published. That first edition consisted of 250 privately published copies of the great manuscript. These copies were published by The Kama Shastra Society, of which Burton himself was a founder. The Kama Shastra Society was created to keep Burton and his peers from being prosecuted and imprisoned by the Society for the Suppression of Vice under the Obscene Publications Act of 1857 and was used by Burton as a method of publishing much of his work over the years. If the society had not been founded, his many endeavors in the field of writing and translation would have been set to the wayside by the popular Victorian society of the time, as Burton, himself, was considered to be less than savory by his peers. His translation and writing often dealt with subjects of an erotic or highly sexual nature which was very counter-culture to the Victorian society of the day.

Some of his works that would otherwise be lost to the world today included a translation of The Book of a Thousand Nights and One Night (Most commonly referred to as The Arabian Nights and considered to be pornography at the time due to sexual content.)and a translation of the Arabic guide called The Perfumed Garden. Sir Richard Burton had written a second translation of the same work which he titled The Scented Garden but this was tragically lost along with several other papers when his widowed wife, Isabel, burned them after his death in October of 1890 from a heart attack. The irony of her destructive action is that Sir Burton had intended this translation to be published after his death as a way of providing for his widow through the proceeds.

The Kama Shastra Society provided for a private publication and distribution of the Kama Sutra to its members thus circumventing the Obscene Publications Act of 1857 because they could not be prosecuted for sharing a private Society publication amongst its members.

It is interesting to note that Sir Burton's work did not become legal in Great Britain until the year 1963, eighty years after its first publication and seventy- three years after Burton's death. What is even more interesting is that a text with absolutely no illustrations was considered so offensive to the British censors.

CAN THE KAMA SUTRA IMPROVE YOUR SEX LIFE?

Things just don't feel the way they used to - sex is starting to seem less like a fun way to spend some quality time and more like a chore, and even masturbating is only mildly exciting. While this happens to a lot of guys - almost all of them, in fact - it is not necessarily a sign that real sexual pleasure is a thing of the past.

The problem is that most men tend to get into a routine. They know what feels good, they know how to please their partner, and it seems natural to do things pretty much the same way every time. But the same old routine can turn boring, and lack of imagination and the same sensations time after time can eventually lead to loss of enjoyment. Even physical loss of penis sensation can occur if an effort is not made to mix things up. Sex therapists and even doctors often recommend the kama sutra for stirring up a stagnating sex life, using these ancient secrets, as well as a mixture of penis-specific vitamins and minerals, to stimulate the senses and open up a whole new range of pleasure.

It is often believed that the kama sutra is some sort of New Age, get-in-touch-with-the-spiritual-side kind of trick, and some men have a hard time believing that a text that is over 2,000 years old can tell them anything they don't already know about sex.

But the truth is that the positions in the kama sutra have been used for centuries for good reason. These positions create a sensual experience that can't be duplicated by a **q**uick grind or a few minutes in the bathroom with a sexy publication or tablet, creating new pressures and new sensations that cannot be experienced in any other way.

HOW CAN THE KAMA SUTRA INCREASE THE EXPERIENCE OF SEXUAL PLEASURE?

There are two basic reasons that the kama sutra works. First of all, the physical side. The skin of the penis, like the skin covering the rest of the body, is subject to all kinds of friction, from rough clothing to rough masturbation to rough sex. Over time, all of this harsh treatment can create a thickened outer layer of dermal tissue, the body's natural response to cell damage. Masturbating or having sex in more or less the same way every time can lead to a callused layer of skin that is less able to respond to sexual stimulation. Therefore, by using the unique positions found in the kama sutra, men can stimulate different areas of the erogenous skin.

Second, the mental side. A large portion of the sexual pleasure experienced by both men and women comes from the brain - people have a huge capacity to visualize what is stimulating, which adds a tremendous amount of excitement to sexual activity. By creating dedicated time and space just for experimenting with the kama sutra, sex becomes an experience, rather than just an act, and the pleasure becomes **infinitely greater.**

The Nirvana

This kama sutra position is ideal for men who lack optimum penis sensitivity. In the Nirvana position, the woman lies on her back, with her arms extended over her head. Her thighs are pressed together, while the man straddles her and penetrates her from this position. This technique is great for both men and women, as it stimulates the clitoris while also exerting gentle pressure on all sides of the penis.

Vitamins and Minerals For Increased Penis Sensation

Treating the penis skin with vitamins and minerals that improve skin tone and moisture and increase nerve receptivity is suggested for men who want to revive their penis sensation. A specially designed penis health formula (most health professionals recommend Man1 Man Oil) containing ingredients such as vitamins A, B5, C, D, and E, as well as antioxidants and natural moisturizers, may increase the suppleness and elasticity of the penis skin, as well as rejuvenating damaged nerve tissue. Having a partner apply a penis crème as part of foreplay can add another sensual dimension to the practice of kama sutra and take the experience of sex to a new level.

Kama Sutra Techniques To Heat Up Any Sex Life

When the words, "Kama Sutra," are uttered, it seems every erogenous zone comes to life and visions of acrobatic and flexible positions come to mind. It's no wonder. The ancient India Sanskrit text is not a sex manual, however. The Kama Sutra is an instructional guide to living one's best life with love and excessive amounts of pleasure. Sounds good, right? Here are a few tips from the 2,400-year-old text that can breathe new life into any sex life.

*Kama Sutra Technique: Churning

Don't be the guy that does the "in and out" which just random thrusts in and out. However, that doesn't mean a man has to hang from a chandelier either. Sometimes, a little twist up can do the trick. Try adding the churn to the mix. Grabbing the penis by the base, move it in small circles inside her vagina. By doing this, a man can not only heighten the pleasure of both partners but also find new hot spots he wasn't aware of.

*Kama Sutra Technique: Take it Down

Trying to stimulate the elusive G-spot with the penis is a gentlemanly and high-level move. However, don't forget the back of the vagina which can yield the especially deep, carnal moans.

While in missionary, instead of thrusting up, thrust downward instead. Either go short and sharp or intermix long, deep strokes with faster ones.

*Kama Sutra Technique: Buffeting

Looking for a way to delay gratification, but also want to keep the raw, lusty, animalistic vibe going? Try buffeting. During thrusting, a man should pull completely out and then thrust back in with a fast, hard stroke. Intersperse it to shake things up or do it, do three short pulses inside and repeat.

*Kama Sutra Technique: Three for the Win

Erogenous zones are all linked, so it's no surprise the stimulating them at the same would lead to a mind-blowing orgasm. Choose three erogenous zones on a partner (lips, ears, nipples, clitoris, etc.) and get to work. A reported winning combo is deep kissing or licking, nipple tweaking, and clitoral stimulation. This also works for men. Feel free to use adult toys to lend a helping hand.

*Kama Sutra Technique: Take Aim

While in missionary, aim the penis to the left or right, keeping firm and continuous pressure on that side of her vagina. Why? One side of the clitoris is almost always more sensitive. Keep the lines of communication open to see which side feels better.

*Kama Sutra Technique: Just an Inch

To switch things up, focus on the second most sensitive spot on a woman, the first inch of the vagina. Using fast, shallow strokes, keeping the penis in (but just barely) will cause those inner nerve endings to go wild. Pair this technique with buffeting for a killer combo.

*Kama Sutra Technique: Rub Her Belly

Okay, it seems a little silly, but rubbing your partner's (if female) belly immediately before orgasm. Why? The area above a woman's pubic bone is highly sensitive. Place both hands flat on her lower abdomen right above her pubic bone. Then move the hands in opposite directions, back and forth across the abdomen. Also, don't stop what's being done to bring her to orgasm in the first place! For male partners, stimulate the perineum in a similar firm pressure, back and forth motion.

With sex this good, a man's penis can get overworked. That's why many men use a specially formulated penis health creme (health professionals recommend Man 1 Man Oil, which has been clinically proven safe and mild for skin) to rejuvenate and restore their penis. Crèmes like these keep the skin soft and supple so chafing and dryness aren't worried and strengthen collagen in the skin with vitamin C. Shea butter and vitamin E seal in hydration while amino acids keep nerve sensitive and strong for a man's every Tantric desire.

ANCIENT ORAL SEXUAL METHODS OF THE KAMA SUTRA

Vatsyayana was a wise man who recognized the sometimes necessary desire for discretion. He knew very well that a sudden outbreak of unexpected pregnancies in the king's harem or of another fellows wife might have some rather serious consequences but as the saying goes "It is better to be a live dog than a dead lion," and sometimes the temptation is just a bit too much.

As the Kama Sutra stated in these clandestine sexual relationships, "No place is as poorly guarded as a harem. And no women more accessible than the king's wives. A determined young man only has to choose how to achieve his ends.

Hidden inside a barrel or disguised as a maidservant, he will easily deceive the casual sentinels and the overworked stewards. He can also try to make himself invisible by using an appropriate potion. But the result is uncertain. The king's wives like to play games with strangers that are forbidden with their husband. The young man and the noble lady are lying against each other, head to tail.

He explores her yoni while her pretty mouth gobbles up his lingam greedily. It is Kalila the crow, the posture of slaves and maidservants, that queens are so fond of." Vatsyayana went on to describe the steps and variations of oral sex in hopes that his pupils might live to enjoy another day.

The Method Of Fellatio In The Kama Sutra

The Kama Sutra describes the act of fellatio in great detail, breaking it down into individual steps. It is described in the following quotes.

"When your lover catches your lingam in her hand and, shaping her lips to an 'O', lays them lightly to its tip, moving her head in tiny circles, this first step is called Nimitta." Nimitta is translated as Touching.

"Next, grasping its head in her hand, she clamps her lips tightly about the shaft, first on one side then the other, taking great care that her teeth don't hurt you. This is Parshvatoddashta." This is called Biting at the Sides.

"Now she takes the head of your lingam gently between her lips, by turns pressing, kissing it tenderly and pulling at its soft skin. This is Bahia-samdansha." This is called the Outer Pincers.

"If next, she allows the head to slide completely into her mouth and presses the shaft firmly between her lips, holding a moment before pulling away, it is Antaha-samdansha." This is translated as the Inner Pincers.

"When she senses that your orgasm is imminent she swallows up the whole lingam, sucking and working upon it with lips and tongue until you spend, this is Sangara." Sangara means Swallowed Whole.

The Method Of Cunnilingus In The Kama Sutra

Of course, one good turn always deserves another, and this was no less true in Ancient Hindu culture. Thus Vatsyayana's Kama Sutra went on to describe the reciprocal act of cunnilingus for the man who wanted to return the favor.

"With delicate fingertips, pinch the arched lips of her house of love very very slowly together, and kiss them as though you kissed her lower lip; this is Adhara-sphuritam." This is rendered the Quivering Kiss.

"Now spread, indeed cleave asunder, that archway with your nose and let your tongue gently probe her yoni, with your nose, lips and chin slowly circling. It becomes Jihva-bhramanaka." Also called the Circling Tongue.

"Let your tongue rest for a moment in the archway to the flower-bowed Lord's temple before entering to worship vigorously, causing her seed to flow. This is Jihva-mardita" or the Tongue Massage.

"Next, fasten your lips to hers and take deep kisses from this lovely one, your beloved, nibbling at her and sucking hard at her clitoris; this is called Chushita." This Chushita is translated as Sucked.

"Place your darling on a couch, set her feet to your shoulders, clasp her waist, suck hard and let your tongue stir her overflowing love-temple. This is called Bahuchushita" or Sucked Hard.

"If the pair of you lie side by side, facing opposite ways, and kiss each other's secret parts using the ten techniques described above, it is known as Kalila." Kalila means Crow.

DISCOVER KAMA SUTRA PLEASURE TO ADD MORE EXOTIC SENSUALITY AND PLEASURE TO YOUR LOVE MAKING

When you think of great sex, you think of the Kama Sutra. The Kama Sutra has become a part of our society in terms of sex because many consider it to be the manual of sex. For great sex, you learn the Kama Sutra because there is a pleasure and then there is the Kama Sutra pleasure.

This Sutra or Teaching came into being thousands of years ago in India but thanks to its spread to the western world, the Kama Sutra has become the standard text on human sexual behavior. Written by Mallanaga Vatsyayana does not devote the entire text to sex. The traditional Kama Sutra is composed of advice on sex, poetry verses, and other prose.

In all, there are seven sections in this Sutra and only the second section is based on sex. It is called On Sexual Union and it details the various sexual positions that make Kama Sutra pleasure such an unbelievable experience.

In this section, you will find various drawings of couples in different positions during sex, as well as oral techniques and advice on how to bite and scratch your partner to give them greater pleasure.

Some of the most popular Sutra pleasure positions are:

•**Widely Open:** The man kneels on the bed and raises the woman's buttocks and thighs so her legs are wrapped around him. As the man thrusts, the woman arches her back and leans backward.

•**Indrani:** This position has the woman lying on her back with her knees bent up to her chest. The man kneels behind the woman and enters her, pulling her up towards him by holding onto her buttocks.

•**The Tigress:** This position has the man lying on the bed with the woman sitting on top of him with her back on towards his face. Often called the Reverse Cowgirl these days.

•**The Congress and the Crow:** This is essentially the 69 position where you are both lying on your sides providing oral sex to each other.

•**Splitting of a Bamboo:** This position has the man on top, with the woman putting one leg up on his shoulder and having the other leg laying down flat. Legs can be alternated during this pleasure position.

These five positions will give you a lot of pleasure and you will see why this book and sensual teachings are considered to be the go-to book for pleasure. Enjoy these Kama Sutra pleasure positions!

DISCOVER KAMA SUTRA PLEASURE TO ADD MORE EXOTIC SENSUALITY AND PLEASURE TO YOUR LOVE MAKING

When you think of great sex, you think of the Kama Sutra. The Kama Sutra has become a part of our society in terms of sex because many consider it to be the manual of sex. For great sex, you learn the Kama Sutra because there is a pleasure and then there is the Kama Sutra pleasure.

This Sutra or Teaching came into being thousands of years ago in India but thanks to its spread to the western world, the Kama Sutra has become the standard text on human sexual behavior. Written by Mallanaga Vatsyayana does not devote the entire text to sex. The traditional Kama Sutra is composed of advice on sex, poetry verses, and other prose.

In all, there are seven sections in this Sutra and only the second section is based on sex. It is called On Sexual Union and it details the various sexual positions that make Kama Sutra pleasure such an unbelievable experience.

In this section, you will find various drawings of

couples in different positions during sex, as well as oral techniques and advice on how to bite and scratch your partner to give them greater pleasure.

Some of the most popular Sutra pleasure positions are:

•**Widely Open:** The man kneels on the bed and raises the woman's buttocks and thighs so her legs are wrapped around him. As the man thrusts, the woman arches her back and leans backward.

•**Indrani:** This position has the woman lying on her back with her knees bent up to her chest. The man kneels behind the woman and enters her, pulling her up towards him by holding onto her buttocks.

•**The Tigress:** This position has the man lying on the bed with the woman sitting on top of him with her back on towards his face. Often called the Reverse Cowgirl these days.

•**The Congress and the Crow:** This is essentially the 69 position where you are both lying on your sides providing oral sex to each other.

•**Splitting of a Bamboo:** This position has the man on top, with the woman putting one leg up on his shoulder and having the other leg laying down flat. Legs can be alternated during this pleasure position.

These five positions will give you a lot of pleasure and you will see why this book and sensual teachings are considered to be the go-to book for pleasure. Enjoy these Kama Sutra pleasure positions!

THE STRATEGIES OF THE ACTUAL KAMA SUTRA

Way back within the second century, Malllanaga Vastyayana gathered one of the world's most legendary books labeled the Kama Sutra. It had been mainly produced to further improve newlyweds love life after a bonded relationship. The Kama Sutra continues to grow to turn out to be just about the most required self-help guides around.

Learning the Book offers an array of tips and hints, many people feel it all about making love and also the postures, yet actually, it's mostly about the build-up to a sexual encounter also, the peacefulness. soon after. Personally coach your self the best way being a lot more seductive lover using the valuable hints and tips, from kissing to intercourse. The book is undoubtedly a huge hit for experimental partners including long-term couples who reQuire to help spice up their intimate sexual contact. The kama sutra will educate you on points regarding each other's body you would not consider possible.

Kama Sutra comprises of two very different meanings. The Kama originated in a Native Indian God Identified as the Kama, It also indicates pleasure or even sensual desire. Sutra meaning solely small books.

This particular guide consists of all sorts of tips and hints, most that'll surprise you, as you could currently feel you understand everything concerning your soul mate's sexual desires as well as physique. You'll find your romantic endeavors becoming considerably more exciting, you'll encounter your love lives going to a new level. No person is the same, everyone has unique likes and dislikes, not simply within the sleeping quarters, The Kama Sutra will cover just about everything regarding everyone's sexual pleasure.

IF you might have ever thought about something connected to the intimacy and also sex with your partner, which puzzles you or have been curious about, the Kama Sutra book has likely discussed it. By using this book to help keep your current love life and romantic endeavors and open a lot of new doors to numerous various sensations.

Using the Kama Sutra guide appropriately and not wanting it to work miracles in one day is very useful to most romantic relationships. It's important to remember it will need greater than a day to get to understand your significant other inside and out. keeping a romantic relationship from going boring can be difficult at all ages, which means Kama Sutra is well suited for anybody of ages young and old. It addresses an array of experimental tricks to try out along with your lover, not all revolving around sex. Mastering specific moves inside the bedroom may be tough, but this specific book is likely to make it easy and exciting to know.

BONING UP ON THE KAMA SUTRA

Between the years of 1990 and 2013, the Internet has become a giant repository for adult educational materials. Now, any guy with a humming Internet connection and a glowing computer screen can research new sex positions to his heart's content, learning all about the Kama Sutra, as well as some new positions that likely hadn't been invented until furniture became just a bit more sturdy. Despite this wealth of information, some men may wonder how much position matters, and others might wonder if certain tricky moves may up the risk of dangerous injuries that require specialized penis care. This article may solve some of those issues for good, at the same time helping men to improve their performance and boost sensitivity in the pertinent parts.

The Case for Tricky Positions

There are times when interesting poses add something special to bedroom antics. Men who are of slightly diminutive size, for example, might enjoy positions that allow them to stand behind their partners as they work, as these poses allow for a deeper sensation of penetration. Similarly, men who are on the slightly larger side of things may enjoy side-by-side positions or those that allow the receiver to control the speed and depth of the movement. Positions that account for these size differences could allow men to please their partners in new ways.

Couples with a long history of intimacy may also enjoy acrobatics, as these new moves allow established couples to experience new sides of their partners, along with new sensations. Incorporating toys or using positions that involve bending, standing or planking could also allow partners to use their muscles in new ways, discovering new erogenous zones they may have passed by with their humdrum routines of the past.

Inherent Dangers

While adding unusual movements could bring some couples intense pleasure, these same movements could also bring a man intense pain without proper precautions. During a sexual escapade, if all is going well, a man's penis is engorged with blood and pulsing with energy. It's a tool that's firm, and it's also a little inflexible. If both couples are moving and the action is less-than-perfectly coordinated, a sudden movement could bring this inflexible penis into contact with a similarly hard bone, toy or piece of furniture. The injuries that can stem from an act like this include:

- Bruises
- Scratches
- Scrapes

•Ruptured penile tissues

Any incident that results in a loud cracking and a sudden change in the appearance of the penis should be treated as a medical emergency, and men need to act accordingly. However, even bruises and cuts might merit medical attention, and the pain can **q**uickly put an end to any hope of intimacy.

The Middle Path

Men don't need to risk the health of their most valuable assets to add a little zip to the bedroom. There are quite a few things both sets of partners can do that could turn up the heat without causing a trip to the emergency room. For example, some couples find that using words during sex adds a little spice to an otherwise routine encounter. By simply describing what is happening now, and what's likely to happen in the future, both partners might become more focused on the action that's unfolding. Similarly, couples who haven't engaged in oral sex or tried incorporating feathers, ice or food into their sex sessions may find that a new experience lies within their reach, with no health risk insight.

Men may also get sex help through the use of a penis health creme. Products like this can nourish sensory cells, so they can transmit signals of pleasure with ease. A well-designed product (most experts recommend Man1 Man Oil) can also help to keep penile skin hydrated, so it's flexible and soft to the touch. A tool like this is destined to respond beautifully in almost any position.

THE KAMA SUTRA OF ROMANCE - ENDLESS POSITIONS OF LOVE!

So, do you think of romance when you hear the term "Kama Sutra?" Some people think of something a little bit more physical, but believe it or not, there are just as many different positions of romance as there are for intercourse.

For those of you who don't know, the Kama Sutra is an ancient text of dozens of sexual positions for loving couples. The Kama Sutra is extremely popular and sought after by lovers who want to add more excitement to their love lives.

But adding real, old-fashioned love to your relationship is one of the best ways possible to improve your sexual and mental satisfaction...and there are endless ways to bring that love into your life. More ways than there are sexual positions in the Kama Sutra!

So the Kama Sutra of Romance, as we will call it, is full of more "positions" to improve your love life than you'll ever find in any sex book. And I guarantee you that the positions you'll discover in the Kama Sutra of Romance will bring much more fulfilling and enduring changes to your love, too.

So, how do you get your hands on a copy and add an endless number of new romantic positions to your love life? Well, believe it or not, the Kama Sutra or Romance can be yours for free...because it's up to you to write it!

That's right: just like every love is unique, so are the different romantic positions that will add new life to your relationship. From romantic dates to honeymoon ideas to pet names, there are endless possibilities... and sometimes, options that are perfect for one love are poison to another.

So as you write your own, remember that the romantic positions that will work for your love aren't the same as anyone else's. Just like the original Kama Sutra, you should never feel guilty about discovering the romantic positions that work best for you and implement them in your love!

And always remember that just because a love relationship doesn't have any physical aspects early on, that doesn't mean that physical attraction and sexual openness can't develop later. The best love is the kind that is nurtured slowly, and the more patient you are, the more likely it is that your relationship will become fulfilling for both partners. Have patience, be willing to try new things, and respect your lover's opinions, and your sexual relationship will develop, as well.

When you look at the most durable, long-lasting and fulfilling romantic relationships in the world, you'll notice that they all have one thing in common: they were developed slowly, over a long period, and the people involved in them were patient. Patience is the common characteristic of every successful relationship, and it's the secret key to uncovering your own Kama Sutra of Romance...and discovering a treasure trove of variety in your romantic life.

UNDERSTANDING THE POSITIONS OF THE KAMA SUTRA

The Kama Sutra is considered a profound scholarly work that delves deeply into human sexuality and its physical expression as well as the psychological aspect of human love. While the original texts were not illustrated, a common misconception, they were very explicit in descriptions and details of a variety of sexual acts and their preludes. Little is known of the text's author, Vatsyayana, but it is conveyed through his writing that the author was of a Hindu religious background and was quite the scholar. It is also evident that the writer was an older individual as conveyed by his vast knowledge of his art. Understanding these points makes the journey into the discovery of the Kama Sutra positions all the more interesting.

What is the Advice in the Kama Sutra?

In looking into the chapter of the Kama Sutra dealing with the art of lovemaking, we early detect that Vatsyayana was a firm believer in the power of foreplay. He advises his readers as follows: "Ardent young men, do not neglect the preliminaries! Endeavor to satisfy your mistress. Listen to her desires. Some men carried away by the power of their desire, forget the prelude, only to be surprised when they have pushed away later! Yet it is such a delight to kiss, to caress, to nibble one another... To explore with your hand or your mouth her body, her breasts, her neck, her belly, down to her innermost curves. Fulfilled, the beloved shall return these kisses and caresses wholeheartedly. No part of the beloved's body should be neglected. Her lover shall make it his duty to discover them, to reveal to his mistress all the pleasure she can receive from them." Vatsyayana knew and understood that a woman needs an emotional attachment to be a great lover and hurried encounters rarely resulted in satisfaction for both parties.

We read of a proliferation of sexual activities, many seeming to require the skills of both a contortionist and an acrobat, later in the chapter including lying down positions (such as Indrani, Churning, Mixture, Yawning, Cobra, Conch and Pestle), sitting positions (including the Black bee, Mare, Swing, Bamboo, Knot, Spare, Tigress and Sharpening), rear-entry positions (with such inventive names such as Inversion, Elephant and Dog), standing poses (including Knee elbow, Stag, Tripod), oral sex (creatively referred to as the Lovemaking of the Crow and noted as "the posture of slaves and maidservants, that queens are so fond of" by Vatsyayana) and the exotic areas of sexual intercourse such as group sexual encounters or the use of Apradravyas, sexual stimulants or aids for the assistance of poorly mated partners. The author went so far as to include an ancient form of male enhancement wherein he advised the reader to "First rub your penis with wasp stings and massage it with sweet oil.

When it swells, let it dangle for ten nights through a hole in your bed, going to sleep each night on your stomach. After this period use a cool ointment to remove the pain and swelling. By this method men... of insatiable sexual appetite, manage to keep their penises enlarged throughout their lives." The method sounds excruciatingly painful and we have no record as to whether Vatsyayana had ever personally tried this particular Apradravya but it is easy to gather from the written work that Vatsyayana was well versed in the sexual arts and positions of the Kama Sutra or had at least made a very thorough study of his subject.

EXTREME KAMA SUTRA POSITIONS!

It's amazing how popular The Kama Sutra has become in recent years. What could it be? Could it be the fact that so many people are now becoming more aware of the need for more adventurous sex life? Or perhaps it's because maybe the western world has a lot to learn when it comes to increasing the level of both pleasure and connection in the bedroom? Whatever it is it sure has had a huge impact on the world and doesn't look like stopping anytime soon!

Some Kama Sutra Positions To Have Fun With

In case you didn't know already, there are hundreds of different kama sutra positions for you and your partner to try in the bedroom. A lot of positions created in ancient times have been modified and we as a western civilization have to give them different names. Some of the more extravagant kama sutra positions include:

•The Waterfall

The waterfall is a fairly difficult position to get into initially and requires a certain level of flexibility, mostly by the woman. You will need a stool for this position. Once you have one, the man should sit down and allow his partner to climb onto, wrapping both legs around his waist. From there the woman should hold onto the inner pelvis region of the man and proceed to rock back as far as she can go, almost touching her head on the ground below her. The man should hold onto her breasts and caress them as she rocks her pelvis in an up and down motion.

This is a very erotic position once you get the hang of it and can create enormous pleasure, especially for the woman as the position she is in allows for the man's penis to press against the upper region of the vagina wall, where a lot of nerve endings appear.

•The Indian Headstand

Again the Indian headstand is a fairly difficult position to get into initially, but once there it's a lot of fun and extremely erotic. It requires the man to be standing and the woman to be taken from behind. The man should firstly hold the upper front on both thighs. From there the woman should move her feet up between his arms resting the backs of her feet on the front shoulders of her partner, all the while keeping her arms straight and her head off the ground. The only part of the body that should be touching the ground is for the woman her hands and the man his feet.

Again it does require a bit of strength mostly by the man to hold her into position, but once there he should proceed to take her from behind.

So there are just a few positions to try out with your partner next time the two of you are feeling like doing something a little more exciting than just the plain old missionary position!

3 KAMA SUTRA POSITIONS THAT EVERY COUPLE SHOULD TRY

The various sexual positions in Kama Sutra are there to help you and your lover enjoy the sexual experience. If both of you have been using the same old positions during lovemaking, is time for a change tonight.

Now, let me share with you 3 mind-blowing Kama Sutra positions that every couple should know and try:

•The Twining Position

This is one of the first few positions mentioned in the Kama Sutra guide. If you only know the Doggy style and missionary, this position is for you. In this position, you and your lover will lie on your side, facing each other. Next, the woman will open her legs slightly, allowing the man to penetrate her. Once the man penetrated her, she can tighten or release the grip on her partner to enjoy different sensations.

•The Clipping Position

In this position, the man will lie down on her back. The woman will sit on top of him and allow him to penetrate her. This position gives the woman 100% control and is great for clitoral stimulation.

•The Pressing Position

This is a very powerful position and when done correctly, can give the lady a mind-blowing g-spot orgasm. The woman will lie on her back and raise her knees to her chin. The man will hold her feet and place them on his shoulders. Next, he holds on to her shins and penetrates her deeply. Remember to start slowly as this position will give the lady intense pleasure.

Varying your sexual positions is important if you want to keep the fire burning in the bedroom. When you always stick to a few old positions, things get boring and sex becomes very dull. Dull sex is never good for your relationship or marriage.

There are many other great sexual positions in the Kama Sutra guide. If you are looking for more Kama Sutra positions to spice up your lovemaking, I strongly urge you to check out the site below.

KAMA SUTRA POSITIONS - ANCIENT SEX TECHNIQUES

The ancient Hindus have a well-developed literary tradition that focuses on the art and science of achieving rewarding sex. The most well-known sex positions can be found in the Kama Sutra. There are several Kama Sutra positions worth recommending in the quest for sexual pleasure: the traditional woman on her back, a man on top position; the man on his back, a woman on top position; and woman with her back to the man. Here are several uniquely named and loosely translated Kama Sutra positions to unleash your most primal desires.

•'Putting On The Sock

' Go ahead try saying it without bursting with laughter or better yet let your imagination run wild. 'Putting on the sock' does not refer to the man covering his penis with a sock. It refers to a very erotic technique with the woman on her back the man sits between her legs and puts his penis at the entrance of her vagina. Slowly caressing her vagina he replaces his fingers with his penis. The continued stroking will leave her incredibly wet, wild and on the verge of an orgasm. The man brings the erotic torture to an end by thrusting into the woman giving her what she truly craves.

•'The Blacksmith's Posture

' In this Kama Sutra position, the woman lies down and drawing her knees to her torso pushing her vagina forward creating a scintillating view. The man then begins the game of teasing her madly by inserting and withdrawing his penis. This Kama Sutra position helps the man maintain a longer erection. Supposedly, this movement imitates the blacksmith who 'draws the hot iron from the fire...' The best thing is that this Kama Sutra position can lead to scorching sex.

•The 'Ostrich's Tail

' With the woman on her back, the man kneels at her feet and then raises her legs until only her head and shoulders remain on the bed or floor. After he enters her she can then put her legs around his head. Her raised legs give the impression of being spread out--like an ostrich's tail. This sensual Kama Sutra position benefits both partners by allowing them to slowing build up to an orgasm.

•The 'Yawning Position

' In this Kama Sutra position, the woman on her back raises and widely spreads her legs as the man eagerly enters her vagina. This position allows the man and woman to share the intimacy of pleasure by gazing into the eyes of each other. The woman can also caress her breasts adding to the visual stimulation.

Of course, I would love to write that these Kama Sutra positions provide earth-shattering orgasms for everyone. The fact is these positions are truly for athletic and adventurous individuals. That's not to say that a modified version wouldn't benefit everyone, so why not give them a try.

KAMA SUTRA POSITION - WOMAN ACTING THE PART AND WORK OF THE MAN

For most of the Kama Sutra positions, man is always at the driving seat, doing his work. But there are some positions in the Kama Sutra manual whereby women can act like men, and help him with his part and work when he is tired.

There is a saying in the Kama Sutra manual, which says: "WHEN a woman sees that her lover is fatigued by constant congress, without having his desire satisfied, she should, with his permission, lay him down upon his back, and assist him by acting his part. She may also do this to satisfy the curiosity of her lover or her desire for novelty." - Kama Sutra

When the woman sees that her lover is tired during intercourse, she can take the initiative and do the thrusting on her own to allow her man to take a rest. The man will appreciate this action by his lover, and will this return a good favor once he has rested enough.

There are 2 ways that a woman can act the part of the man. The first is when during congress she turns around, and gets on the top of her lover, in such a manner as to continue the congress, without obstructing the pleasure of it; and the other is when she acts the man's part from the beginning.

The Kama Sutra also states that while the woman is acting the part of the man, she can say something that has a similar meaning to this sentence: "I was laid down by you, and fatigued with hard congress; I shall now, therefore, lay you down in return."

When the woman is acting the part of the man and feels tired, she should place her forehead on his and take rest. Upon seeing this, the man should turn around and continue to do the thrusting again.

IMPROVING YOUR RELATIONSHIP WITH KAMA SUTRA POSITIONS

These days the kama sutra book is a very well known guide to the practices of making love all over the world. It was originally written in the 8th Century B.C. and has been used ever since as a tool for improving loving partners' sex lives as well as providing the famous karma sutra positions.

However, the kama sutra is more than just a list of sexual positions; it is a guide to creating an all-round better relationship with your partner in a way that transcends the physical. The premise behind the kama sutra book is that by using a variety of kama sutra positions as well as following the other tips you will learn to think just as much about your partner's pleasure as your own.

So what are some of the other aspects of the karma sutra? Well, there is a strong emphasis on cleanliness so, before delving straight into the kama sutra positions you should take the time to clean each other in a shared shower or bath. This process can be part of your foreplay and the kama sutra book recommends that patients should be shown and that you should feel thoroughly clean so that there will be no distraction during the act of lovemaking.

Then, according to the karma sutra, you should begin the foreplay in earnest. The idea of patience and taking one's time is again emphasized in the karma sutra positions. Also, spend as much time kissing, caressing and breathing on various parts of the body (not only mouths and genitals) as you would in actual penetrative sex.

Once you feel you have both built up enough tension and excitement you can begin the full act of penetrative sex. Although the karma sutra sexual positions are the most famous aspect of the karma sutra book, most people are not familiar with the vast majority of them. There are scores of different forms and positions, each one providing the participants with different types of stimulation.

After both, you and your partner have reached orgasm the kama sutra stresses that your lovemaking is not over and you should make an effort to continue the sensual atmosphere and perhaps cool down together with a shower.

It is important to remember that by being aware that this act is more than the kama sutra positions and if you take your time to enjoy each aspect of the karma sutra, you and your partner will lead a healthier and more enjoyable life together.

AMAZING KAMA SUTRA POSITIONS - THE FUSION, POSSESSION, AND FACE TO FACE

Kama Sutra Position 1 - The Fusion

In this position, the man sits down, tilting his body slightly backward, supporting it by bracing his hands on the bed on each side of his body. The legs may be stretched or bent, depending on the partner's comfort. The heads of both partners should be relaxed. The woman assumes the active role on this occasion, passing her legs over her lover and supporting herself by bracing her arms behind her body.

To be successful in this position, stimulation must be intense, since during penetration this position prevents manual contact and contact of the mouths of the partners.

The woman sets the rhythm and establishes the genital encounter with a very marked motion. It is essential to have the clitoris take full advantage of the impacts with her lover's body to maintain the excitement until the moment she decides to explode with pleasure, provided her lover keeps the rhythm with a good erection.

The look is a fundamental component, but so is essential and provocative communication, since erotic words provide a very strong sexual charge to the love act. Both resources (looks and words) can be unbelievable weapons used to enjoy this position and achieve a complete "fusion".

Kama Sutra Position 2 - Possession

As its name indicates, this position is captivating and has a certain degree of suggestion, especially for the woman. The man can use all his sexual magnetism and enjoy his energy in this posture.

The woman lies on her back with her legs open, waiting for her partner to penetrate her, while he sits down and holds her by her shoulders to regulate the motion. Their legs become intertwined sensually and pleasantly.

The male organ penetrates and withdraws, deviating its movement downward since the body of the woman is slightly higher than the body of the man. He can then explore the woman's G spot and all of her genital area to give his partner everything she loves.

Kama Sutra Position 3 - Face to Face

This is the most classic and universal position known in the art of making love. It provides a lot of security for couples in which the woman needs the man's bodily, sexual, and emotional protection.

The state of being face to face makes for a large number of variations to this position, which makes it an attractive and exciting one. The mobility of the hands, the closeness of the faces, and the comfort of the bodies are some of the advantages that made it famous.

The lovers should not fear trying new types of the contract during the love act in this position. She can touch her mate's glutei and anal areas. He can rub her clitoris or allow her to do it herself. The legs of both partners may be closer together to create a certain degree of difficulty in the penetration.

HOT KAMA SUTRA POSITIONS - THE SCREW, THE AMAZON, AND THE EASY CHAIR

Kama Sutra Position 1 - The Screw

Nothing is more advisable to a woman who finds it difficult to reach orgasm than assuming positions that press on the clitoris while the vagina is penetrated. Orgasm always comes in this position, and multiple experiences of pleasure become concrete and unforgettable feelings for the woman.

She lies down by the edge of the bed and places her flexed legs to one side of her body (each woman will know which side is most comfortable for her). This enables her to keep the clitoris trapped between the best allies she has to reach the prized orgasm - the labia or her vagina.

The woman can contract and relax that entire region, while the man, kneeling in front of her, penetrates her softly. To turn this position into a true delicacy, it is suitable for the man, while penetrating her, to caress her breasts and for the woman to groan with pleasure to arouse her partner.

Kama Sutra Position 2 - The Amazon

This position puts the woman in an active position. She places herself on top of the man and sets the rhythm of the sexual relation by bracing her feet on the floor. It is ideal for active women who are a bit domineering and like to set the sexual rhythm in a relationship.

For the man, this is an extraordinary experience

because in this position he can incorporate the yin energy, which is more passive, and also, be able to relax in the course of the sexual act. In turn, he can touch her breasts and pull the hair on his mate while she moves.

The visual angle made possible by this variation is one of the most exciting angles for the man since he can see close at hand each thrust he performs on his partner. And the woman will get much pleasure from the idea of knowing that she is in control of the sexual act and the woman knows it.

Kama Sutra Position 3 - The Easy Chair

Leaning on a big, comfortable cushion or pillow, the man sits with his legs flexed and a bit open. The woman sits comfortably on the space he's formed with his body. In this position, the protective feelings of both partners come to the fore.

Assisted by his arms and hands, the man finds the satisfactory point of encounter for both and places his partner on his erection, controlling the sexual rhythm.

Her legs are braced on the shoulders of her mate, who has his head trapped and wrapped between her thighs. The man can touch her clitoris while forcefully grabs her by her waist.

The distance between the faces and the daring aspect of this proposal endow this position with an extremely sensual quality.

TOP KAMA SUTRA POSITIONS - THE TRAPEZE, THE MIRROR OF PLEASURE, AND THE DRAGONFLY

Kama Sutra Position 1 - The Trapeze

The man sits with his legs open and his partner, on top of him, opens up to slow penetration, feeling fulfilled and giving herself up to her lover to be complemented.

The man takes the woman by the wrists while he feels an overwhelming joy toward her. Then he leans back, relaxing slowly until he falls back completely. It is important for the woman to remain relaxed and to give herself up to the strength of her lover, who draws her in with his arms and engages in the powerful thrusts needed for the act of lovemaking.

The position combines several movements. It requires agility and a relaxed surrender on the part of the woman, and strength and skill on the part of the man. Both balance and complement each other.

This position is ideal for changing the routine and for experiencing new emotions.

Kama Sutra Position 2 - The Mirror of Pleasure

The woman lies on her back and lifts her legs in a vertical position while her breathing betrays the joy of showing her wet and longing parts to her partner. She then lets him hold her legs, with her partner kneeling at the end of her body and propping his other arm on the floor. The man penetrates her, subdues her, and controls her, varying the direction of the penetration and the opening of the legs.

Their faces can't get near each other and the man's hands can do very little in this position, which generates an extremely arousing anxiety. The two bodies run the race together to reach orgasm, bestowing on each other the most varied gestures of pleasure, sensuality, affection, and eroticism.

Kama Sutra Position 3 - The Dragonfly

To perform the sexual act in this position, the partners must lie on their sides in a flexible and comfortable place, such as a bed or a sofa. The woman lies on her side with her back turned to her partner, and he mounts her from the back. This way, the bodies fit each other in a position that is ideal for very affectionate couples who enjoy demonstrating the tenderness they feel toward each other.

With a bit of skill combined with much excitement, the woman takes her flexed outer leg and places it on the man's coccyx, thus opening the door to pleasure. The man penetrates her by using his lover's leg as an erotic lever bracing on the support of his hip.

The flattering words the man can whisper in his partner's ear, because it is so close to his mouth, provide the perfect compliment to achieve the utmost delight, in addition to ardent kisses. The woman, upon just listening to him, lets herself be taken over by the rhythm of his kisses, while she shows her lover all the affects his potency has on her through her expressions of intense pleasure.

Penetration goes halfway, which is why the pleasure is enhanced by the desire to make penetration deep and cause the explosion of the most exciting orgasm.

TOP KAMA SUTRA POSITIONS - THE SLEEPY WOMAN, THE SURPRISE, AND THE MEDUSA

Kama Sutra Position 1 - The Sleepy Woman

The woman lies on her side and the man mounts her from the back to penetrate her. She stretches a leg backward and wraps it around his waist. This position is ideal for well-endowed men who always had experiences in the traditional position, and for very flexible women who want to place their whole body at the disposal of their mate.

Additionally, it fulfills several longings of fantasy-driven minds. First of all, she is in front of him and at the same time has access to his face and neck, and he has access to her face and neck. Secondly, he has comfortable access to her clitoris and can touch and feel the breasts of his lover.

Kama Sutra Position 2 - The Surprise

In this position, the man must be standing up to grab the woman from behind, penetrating her, and at the same time take her by the hips in a sensual manner and with a certain degree of domination. She relaxes her whole body and places her hands on the floor in an attitude of surrender and of confidence in her partner. The man "surprises" the woman from behind, setting the erotic rhythm almost completely.

For her, pleasure is concentrated because of the opening angle of the vagina, which, being narrow, provokes a very intense, pleasant sensation. For him, the most powerful sensation expands upward from the glans, which comes into and out of the vagina at will and caresses the clitoris in the most daring moves as it comes out. Also, the man's visual field covers her anus, her buttocks, and her back, zones that are very erogenous for many people. The domination exerted by the man on the woman together with her complete relaxation may foster playfulness in the man, who while seducing his lover can play around with her anus. If she already knows the experience, the woman may approach the sensation of pleasure caused by her lover's anal penetration.

This position is ideal for those who love the most savage and primitive forms of sexual intercourse.

Kama Sutra Position 3 - The Medusa

The partners should kneel on a comfortable surface, though not as soft as a bed. In this position, the man surrenders to the woman's will. She descends on his penis and introduces it into her vagina whenever she wishes. Before penetration, they may kiss, rub each other's breasts, hug, caress each other's back, and place the glans in her vagina and rub it against the clitoris, creating a pleasant and very different sensation, an almost unique one. After being very much desired, the penetration will come with infinite pleasure at the end.

In the course of the love act, if he can't surrender patiently to her moves, he'll be able to set the rhythm by grabbing her by the waist and drawing her body to his.

Since the partners are face to face, this offers the exciting opportunity to observe each other, rejoice together, talk, and kiss each other on the mouth until achieving the much-desired orgasm.

THE KAMA SUTRA AND MASTURBATION: FIVE PIECES OF ANCIENT WISDOM ABOUT PLEASURE

The is no sensual text **q**uite like the Kama Sutra for increasing pleasure and intimacy. While the Kama Sutra doesn't touch on masturbation outright, it does touch on genital touching in general and is very sex-positive. While written for couples, there is a lot of information and guidance that can be applied to self-love, so much in fact that it was easy to find five ways the Kama Sutra elevates masturbation. Here are five of the biggest game-changers the ancient text delivers for an extraordinary experience with the self.

*Open the Mind and Heart

Like any person searching for enlightenment, it's important to have an open mind and heart. Masturbation is a simple function, but it doesn't have to be routine or boring. By approaching the sensual art of self-pleasure in the same way a man would pleasuring a lover, he can find a greater sense of pleasure and ecstasy.

*Remove Guilt from Self-Pleasure

Unlike other sacred traditions that villainize bodily pleasure, the Kama Sutra celebrates it. Sex is a healthy activity that honors the body. It both relaxes the nerves and stimulates blood flow around the body. Aside from physical benefit, intimacy with the self is a beautiful thing and removes societal conditioning like blame, shame, and guilt from sexual urges and pleasure. Once the mind is free of guilt, it can truly explore all the goodies the Kama Sutra provides masturbation.

This removal of guilt allows a man to draw-out and enjoy the process of self-pleasuring. They can relax and go slower, which is not only good mentally, but physically as well. Men who utilize a "death grip" or stroke fast and furious are more likely to cause tiny tears in the skin that lead to scarring or decreased sensation. This acceptance of masturbation as a positive and healing act keeps the penis in tip-top shape for intimacy with a partner as well.

•Embrace Diversity

The Kama Sutra has no shortage of positions for couples to try. From the Padlock to the Rocking Horse, there are tons of ways to enjoy intimacy with a partner. Applying this to self-gratification, one can experience new solo sensations by experimenting with hand positions, pleasure aids, different lubricants, different locations for masturbation, and even exploring other erogenous zones in tandem with masturbation.

Guys who use their left hands should switch to the right for all the new feels. Use a penis sleeve instead with lube to upgrade self-pleasure to exciting heights. Masturbate in the shower instead of only in bed. Maybe it's time to switch things up and stroke with the left hand while stimulating the perineum with the right. If the Kama Sutra teaches anything, it's to experiment and explore!

•Get Tantric

Tantra is a game-changer and is all over the Kama Sutra. Using tantra, men are encouraged to enjoy the journey (of a thousand strokes) rather than stroking fast and orgasming in under ten seconds. Tantra engages the mind and prolongs the pleasure. Here's how to implement some tantric methods when masturbating:

•Fantasize before even touching the penis. Use the mind rather than pictures or movies.

•Slowly undress and pay attention to the feeling of air on the genital area.

•Using a lubricant, slowly stroke the penis while continuing the internal fantasy.

•When the release is near, slow down or completely

stop stroking the penis until ready to begin again.

•Repeat until ready for release.

Slowing down the process not only makes the penis more sensitive in general but also intensifies the orgasm. It's next-level masturbation.

•Keep it Clean

It's only natural that a text about sex includes properly cleaning and anointing (a fancy word for moisturizing) the body before and after sex. Men who solo play should clean up with a gentle wash and thorough rinse. Afterward, air dry or pat dry the penis with a soft towel. Then, reward the penis by applying a penis health creme (health professionals recommend Man 1 Man Oil, which has been clinically proven safe and mild for skin). to keep it protected, smooth, and always ready for action. Products like this not only keep skin soft and supple but also prevent peripheral nerve damage and keep bacteria at bay ensuring he is always prepared for pleasure.

UNVEILING THE SECRETS OF THE KAMA SUTRA

When it comes to The Kama Sutra, more specifically the sexual positions of The Kama Sutra, most people tend to shy away from the more extravagant methods that have huge potential to create a lot of pleasure for both people in a relationship. So what are some of these positions?

Lying Down Positions

Many positions require both people to lie down. Some of these positions you may have already found yourself doing in the past. Here's a couple of them:

The "Flower in Bloom" is where the woman clasps

onto her buttocks with the palms of her hands, while spreading her thighs wide and digging her heels beside her hips, while the man caresses her breasts at the same time.

The "Vyomapada"(more commonly known as the sky foot) is where the woman grabs onto her feet and pulls them up to her hair, whilst laying on her back. This requires some practice and also a bit of flexibility too!

The "Monkey" seems a little weird at first but can create a lot of pleasure for both people. It's when the woman grabs her ankles and raises them skyward whilst the man is on top kissing and 'slapping' her breasts. Try it out, it's great fun, even if it's just for a laugh!

Standing Positions

Standing positions are the most erotic of all positions. Some of them are very extravagant but extremely pleasurable at the same time. Here's a couple for you to try:

The "Avalambitaka" requires the man to be standing up against the wall, holding her underneath the thighs, which she squeezes up against his sides. She then pushes against the wall back and forth, while the man suspends her.

The "Traivikrama" is where the man lifts one of the woman's legs so it is clasped behind his knee. She has her arms around his neck and he makes love to her. This one is very erotic, give it a try!

The "Janukurpara" requires the man to put his elbows under her knees, clasp onto her buttocks and lift her, while she hangs onto his neck. This one has the potential to create an enormous amount of pleasure for both people.

When it comes to positions of The Kama Sutra, there are too many to try. I mean, you've probably already tried many, so make it your goal to only try some of the extravagant ones because they are a lot of fun for the both of you!

KAMA SUTRA: THE BIGGEST MISCONCEPTION

In the western hemisphere and the majority of countries in the eastern hemisphere, the Kama Sutra is seen as a guide for love-making and different things to try in the bedroom with your significant other.

While the Kama Sutra does offer advice on the sexual union of a married couple, this is only a small part of a very large ancient Sanskrit text, creating a huge misconception. Very few people in countries where the Kama Sutra is not regarded as a sacred, religious text don't realize the value of the text when it comes to marriage, relationships, courting and the laws of attraction. Before any relationship advice of any type is given, the text gives a discussion on life's major priorities and the act of gaining knowledge.

Fortunately, the knowledge of just a few facts regarding the Kama Sutra can help debunk the biggest, most common misconception about its contents.

The Seven Parts

The Kama Sutra is divided into seven different parts, only one of which discusses sexual union. The other six include an introduction, how to get a wife, conduct surrounding a wife, the behaviors of men and women, dating and choosing a spouse, and how to attract a spouse.

Through these seven parts, Kama is fully explored. The Kama, or aesthetic and erotic please, I one of the four goals of life. The other three include Dharma (a life of virtue), Artha (prosperity), and Moksha (spiritual liberation).

Courtship

Six chapters of the Kama Sutra are dedicated to the art of dating, or courtship. The writings are ancient, so you won't find advice on creating a good matrimonial site profile, but it does offer timeless pieces of advice essential to finding a *q*uality life partner.

The ancient writers advise how to look for a steady partner, make money to support a relationship, and how to rekindle the romance with a lost lover.

Law of Attraction

To find a lasting mate, it's important to know how to attract the right type of person into your life. You need to have compatible personalities in addition to the initial physical attraction to each other. Two chapters of the Kama Sutra are dedicated solely to advise on how to improve physical attraction between you and your potential spouses, and, once the attraction is established, how to spark a sexual power.

Obtaining Wives & Marriage

Five chapters alone are dedicated to the steps and theories involved in obtaining a wife, and even more talk about the relationship with a wife once the marriage is established.

The ancient advice involves how to get a girl to relax around you and how to make her yours forever. Even in modern times where dating is much more casual and matrimonial sites can be used to introduce and ease the initial awkwardness between a potential couple, this advice is timeless.

HOW PRACTICAL ARE THE POSES MENTIONED IN THE KAMA SUTRA?

The Kama Sutra is a love manual written by Vatsyayana. The book reflects the liberal atmosphere that existed in India before the advent of the Muslims. The book written in the 2-5 century AD is in Sanskrit.

Vatsyayana was a high caste Indian and he must have been very fit and athletic. For as a first step to practice all the poses as enunciated in the Kama Sutra -physical fitness is of paramount importance. Some of the poses are not for men and women who are not supple and flexible. Despite being unable to practice all the poses the Kama Sutra will still awaken your inner sexual voice.

However, bear in mind that the positions described in the Kama Sutra are actually to be tried as a sort of fun. Most likely a lot of them are not practicable and require you to be supple and fit to a great degree, which a lot many of us are not. Thus these poses should just be read and played to a degree with your partner. But some poses if faithfully followed are truly innovative and increase sexual enjoyment.

Remember that the sex act is a total union of men and women in both body and mind. For the mind, you will need intellect and for the body, you need to be in unison with your partner to achieve fulfillment. Hence do read the Kama Sutra but practice only what you and your partner can faithfully achieve. After all, the sexual pleasure is supposed to originate from the meeting of lingam and yoni (male organ and female organ). The Kama Sutra describes nearly 84 poses. But do not get confused in trying to practice all of them. An attempt to do all the poses may leave you in a mess.

The Kama Sutra is to be read with your partner and the effect is to heighten pleasure. From that aspect, it is a monumental work. But keep your counsel otherwise you could pull a muscle and strain yourself.

Bear in mind that sexual reproduction is central to evolution. Darwin's theory and the survival of the species are related to a strong sexual instinct. It is this sexual instinct that Vatsyayana refers to in his book. It is not a religious manual but clinical work. Read it for knowledge and wisdom.

KAMA SUTRA SEX POSITIONS PICTURES - HOW TO FIND THEM ONLINE

Kama Sutra is perhaps the most popular sex manual ever. There are tons of related products available in a different format (video, book, and audio), ranging from few to hundreds of dollars. However, since it is a public domain work, the information is scattered throughout the World Wide Web. With little patience and few tricks, you can find Kama Sutra positions pictures easily:

•Google Search Engine

With a search engine, you can locate any information easily with the right search term. I highly recommend Google as it provides the best and most accurate result. However, do not expect to type "Kama Sutra" into the search box and get the sex positions pictures you want. It doesn't work this way. You need to be as specific as possible to ensure the best results. Here's how:

•Specify the position: the common sex positions illustrated in Kama Sutra are: Cowgirl, Reversed Cowgirl, Missionary, Lotus, Water Embrace, Doggy, Clasping, Widely Opened, Tao, and Ananga Ranga.

•Do not limit to text search. Utilize Google's image, books, and video search function.

•Wikipedia

Wikipedia has a dedicated page on the "List of sex positions". The positions explained are similar to the ones in Kama Sutra. The page has detailed explanations and pictures of various sexual positions. At the end of the page, you can find links to recommended sites on similar subjects.

Besides, in section 1, we've specified some of the common positions. You can search for the related terms on Wikipedia and its recommended websites.

•Wikimedia Common

Another wonderful place to locate Kama Sutra positions pictures is Wikimedia Common. It's an online portal that published public domain and freely-licensed educational content.

The best Kama Sutra positions will not help you if you have a small penis.

KAMA SEX SUTRA - THE DIFFERENT KINDS OF EMBRACES IN KAMA SUTRA THAT CAN TURN YOU WILD

In the Kama Sutra manual, there are various sex positions and techniques that you can explore with your lover. Kama sex Sutra is one of the most sought after theories by couples who wish to explore more into sexual positions and techniques.

In the Kama Sutra manual, there are different ways that a couple can embrace to maximize the penetration and fulfillment level during sexual intercourse.

When both you and your lover are standing, 2 types of embraces can take place, they are:

•The woman clings to the man as a creeper twines

round a tree, bends his head down to hers with the desire of kissing him, embraces him, and looks lovingly towards him, it is called the "twining of a creeper".

•The woman places one of her feet on the foot of her lover, and the other on one of his thighs, passes one of her arms around his back, and the other on his shoulders, makes slightly the sounds of singing and cooing, and wishes, as it were, to climb up him in order to have a kiss, it is called an embrace like the 'climbing of a tree'.

There are also different types of embraces that you can use with your lover while both of you are lying down on the bed:

•The man presses the jaghana or middle part of the woman's body against his own, and mounts upon her to practice, either scratching with the nail or finger, biting, or striking, or kissing, the hair of the woman being loose and flowing, it is called the "embrace of the jaghana".

•One of two lovers presses forcibly one or both of the thighs of the other between his or her own, it is called the "embrace of thighs"

•Either of the lovers touches the mouth, the eyes and the forehead of the other with his or her own, it is called the "embrace of the forehead".

These are just some of the embraces in the Kama Sutra manual that you can use in the bedroom to enhance the intimacy with your lover.

KAMA SUTRA PRODUCTS

When you think of great sex, the first thing that comes to your mind is Kama Sutra. The Kama Sutra came into existence thousands of years ago in India but very soon it was spread all across the globe. Sutra or Teaching Written by Mallanaga Vatsyayana is a collection of guidance on sex, poetry verses, and other styles. It is the oldest and most noteworthy of a group of texts generally known as Kama Shastra. The idea behind this particular Sutra is that by using the various positions mentioned in the book and follows the tips you learn to think much about the satisfaction of your partner as your own. Kama Sutra has become the typical transcript of human sexual manners.

Nowadays you can find lots of nice products that you can use to make your night special and memorable. These are some of the things which are created in perfect accord with today's interest in the well-being of spirit, mind, and body. The motive behind those lust accelerating range of products is to make love even better. They are focused on helping loving couples create fantastic experiences of intimacy and tenderness. Through such closeness, physically and emotionally healthier human beings come out, who in turn out to be more capable to give love to the world. These things have always helped affectionate couples practice a closer level of relationship and enjoy making love. Some of those amazing items are massage oils, luxury bathing gels, bedside boxes, etc. These are specially created to bring people closer and to help heal the sores that were slashing one's world apart.

If you want to create a sensual experience with your partner, go for the body paints. These body paints are available in various flavors, such as delightful chocolate, vanilla, tempting strawberry, intoxicating champagne or sweet honey. All you need to do is just dip the paintbrush or your fingers into the rich and thick body paint and apply it on your lover's body to create your masterpiece and then enjoy the sweet taste of their skin. Or you can also opt for pleasurable balms. Simply apply a small amount of the balm to any of your desired pleasure points and enjoy the exciting sensation and joy in this licky treat. Just bring up the warmth in your closest moments with the love of your life.

LOVE MAKING TIPS TO PRACTICE YOUR KAMA SUTRA TECHNIQUES

Couples always seek out to the Kama Sutra manual to learn more about sexuality, new sexual positions, and techniques. With the help of the Kama Sutra manual, most couples can bring their sexual enjoyment to a brand new height. But that is not all, the sky is the limit.

Kama Sutra's positions and techniques that are taught in the manual are too technical. I will not deny that when you and your lover try out some new positions in the bedroom, there will be a chance that both of you will enjoy it a lot. But what is after that? There will come a time whereby you and your lover will most probably try all those "new" positions before.

It is especially true when a couple has been together for a long while and finds that sexual intercourse is turning very routine and plain boring. This will greatly affect the mood to have sex.

Therefore it is important to be a little creative and innovative in the bedroom to once a while creates the element of surprise for your lover. There are plenty of new ideas out there whereby you can use in the bedroom to increase the intimacy between you and your lover.

For example, do you know that there is an item in your freezer that will send shivers up and down your lover's body in a very surprising way? Or something that you can use in your toiletry bag which doubles as an amazing sex toy?

I bet that most of you do not know about the ideas above, which is why you are missing out on a lot of ideas that can enhance your sex life to a more amazing and fulfilling experience.

PREPARING FOR THE TRUE KAMA SUTRA

The Kama Sutra was written in India between the third and fifth centuries, and its authorship is attributed to the scholar Vatsyayana. It combines Taoist sexual techniques gathered from Chinese bedroom books with the seduction methods described by the Roman poet Ovid, although the Kama Sutra places more emphasis on love (distinguishing it from desire and passion) than did Ovid and the Chinese. Vatsyayana repeatedly interrupts his descriptions of sexual techniques or seduction to insist that the rules do not apply to people in love, who only have to let themselves go and be led by instinct.

Most people associate the Kama Sutra simply with multiple positions in which to perform the sexual act, a mixture of pornography and acrobatics. In the Orient, the true meaning of the Kama Sutra lies very far from this purely gymnastic idea.

From both the perspective of the Tao of love and that of Tantra, every sexual union is sacred and reproduces the ultimate act of creation: the union of the male and female cosmic principles, a union that is the cause of the created and manifest universe. Sexual contact, no matter how trivial it may seem, is sacred and cosmic, even when those who experience such sexual contact are aware of this.

The Kama Sutra teaches a series of asanas, which are yoga positions that have ritualistic meaning. Its purpose is to "divinize" the couple and their sexuality. Without this spiritual component, the Kama Sutra loses its ritualistic meaning.

The aim of the positions is not only to experience sensual voluptuousness but also to facilitate meditation as a couple. Some positions enable them to prolong the sexual union for up to two hours without the need to move much, so as not to disturb the internalization of the divine sexual act. Often the comfort level is such that it allows a complete physical and mental relaxation that will lead them to various states of awareness.

Asanas also promote exchanges of magnetic and vital energies and facilitate the control of ejaculation. In this regard, Tantra disregards, at least at the beginning, the position most often used in the west, commonly known as the missionary position, in which the man lies on top of the woman. This position, according to the scholars, does not facilitate seminal control.

A COMPARISON OF THE PERFUMED GARDEN AND THE KAMA SUTRA

Comparisons are always odious but sometimes they can stimulate the thinking process and lead an intellectual further on his path of seeking knowledge. The Perfumed Garden and the Kama sutra are two works that concern the sexual side of human life. Both were written in a bygone age and have stood the test of time.

The Kama sutra written in Sanskrit is the older book having been complied in the 2nd century about the Julian calendar on the Christian Common Era. It probably dates to 101-200. The author of the Kama sutra is supposed to be Vatsyayana. However, we know very little about the author except that he was a Brahmin. The purpose of writing the book was to show a way to the realization of God.

The perfumed garden, on the other hand, was written in Arabic and came much later. The book is credited to Sheik Nefzaouj and was compiled in the 16th century. Not much is known of the Sheik either. It has no pious intentions like the Kama Sutra but is written with the idea of arousing sensual pleasure. However, both books were translated by Richard Burton an English man and we must remain forever indebted to him for his painstaking effort. The western world has not produced any ancient erotic manuals, perhaps because of the straight jacket approach of Christianity and the earlier puritan approach. But the eastern manuals recognized the sexual side of the man and the result is two great masterpieces of erotic literature.

Both the books though dealing with sex have followed different approaches. The perfumed garden is more like a storybook with nearly 22 stories as part of the text. These are erotic stories and the effort of the sheik is to integrate them with the main text and bring out the essence of the sexual nature of man. They also serve as a guide for attaining extreme bliss- for one cannot deny the fact that the sex act by itself is the most potent form of pleasure in the world.

Vatsyayana's Kama Sutra, on the other hand, is a relatively clinical book. The book represents a different culture and is closely entwined with religion. Hindu philosophy has recognized tantra and sex as a form of achieving god and the authors the main purpose is an exposition of this aspect of the Hindu religion. The book reads more like a manual or treatise and reading it one can glean that the book's intentions are different from the book written by Sheik.

As per the original translation of Burton in 1883 the Kama sutra has 1250 verses distributed over 36 chapters which are further divided into 7 parts. The book deals with all aspects of sex including types of women, the sexual poses, diets for rejuvenation and a host of other sexual matters. It is a monumental work and one can glean a lot of knowledge from this book.

The perfumed garden, on the other hand, is pure erotica and reads more like a fairy tale book. It engrosses the readers with their stories. Interspersed with the stories is good advice on all matters relating to sex. Over the centuries both books have been read and reread any number of times and are a source of intense gratification to most readers. It is a moot point that most works on the sexual side of man's relationship with a woman have emerged from the orient. I will recommend reading both books -nothing can be better than that.

DISCOVERING THE KAMA SUTRA

The Kama Sutra was intended to be a guide on basic human sexuality. It was a guide for a man and a wife to have a successful marriage and a healthy sex life, but today we commonly use it exclusively as a sexual position manual. When you flip through the book you may see large sections of text, but also a lot of pictures. Read this article and you will be able to read your Kama Sutra with ease!

The Text

The text of this book is primarily a happy marriage guide, as many of the guides, we have today. This book helps men and women look attractive and suggests certain foods and scents attract lovers. It talks about how to choose a wife and figure out male and female roles. It also offers advice to a man or woman who has angered their spouse and wishes to make up, and it even advises how to keep your friendship alive with your earlier lovers as well as your spouse. The Kama Sutra also gives practical advice on obtaining money and managing a household.

The Pictures

The sexual instruction section can be very confusing and intimidating when first looking at it, but if you read the instructions it isn't as scary. These positions are supposed to increase the pleasure for both parties as well as maximize the spiritual/intimate connection that sex is supposed to reinforce. The instructions and commentary tell you exactly how to perform the positions without hurting anyone, and encourages you to create your positions once you have mastered their positions. The Kama Sutra also gives suggestions on certain toys, fragrances and foods you can incorporate into your sexual experience. Now the Kama Sutra is meant to be read as an ancient Hindu Text, so not all the information will apply to you if you do not follow the religion, but there is a lot of sexual advice to be gleaned by the people who knew what they were talking about!

Now that you know what the Kama Sutra contains, you can go buy it without any hesitation!

KAMA SUTRA ORGASMS - BEST POSITIONS TO GIVE HER ORGASMS ECSTASY

Every man will want to get their partners to achieve orgasms while making love. When she does not reach orgasm during lovemaking, you will feel down and lousy. But with the help of the Kama Sutra, you will be able to discover some of the classic positions that will send both of you to climax.

•The Doggy Position

This is a classic and highly stimulating position for couples to enjoy during lovemaking. The woman will go down on all fours, taking her weights on her forearms. The man will kneel behind her and penetrate her from the back. The position is very pleasurable for both partners as the deep penetration will not only stimulate the vaginal walls, but also the g-spot. However, some women may feel demeaning if asked to adopt this position. Therefore it will be wise for you to communicate with your partner beforehand and make sure that she is OK with it.

•The Lotus Position

This is an extremely intimate and passionate position which I will strongly encourage you to try it out with your partner. The man sits with both his legs crossed on the bed. The woman will sit on him with both her legs wrapping around his waist. He will then help her to move her hips with his hands and can also caress her breasts with his mouth and stroke her buttock. Once the man has ejaculated, the couple should stay in this position and embrace each other at least for a few minutes, to enjoy the passionate, satisfying, intimate moment.

These 3 positions that I have shared with you are considering the best in the Kama Sutra manual according to my opinion. You may not feel the same.

FEMALE KAMA SUTRA - SEXUAL SATISFACTION FOR WOMEN

Its all about what women want out of sexual relationships. The kama sutra talks [actually preaches] about the satisfaction of the males in sexual unions without the female satisfaction being considered. Today, females have taken their sexual destinies into their own hands and are no longer docile in sexual matters. Women have started talking about what they want out of sex and lovemaking and the more daring among the female folk have started getting what they want out of sex and sexual relationships. More women are walking out from relationships that fail to satisfy them sexually and moving into better sexually satisfying relationships. Lovemaking ought to be enjoyed by all parties to it and not one party to the exclusion of the other.

The agitation for sexual satisfaction for women is a healthy development and discerning men are now realizing that sex does not end with their ejaculation or orgasm. Besides, what manner of sexual satisfaction will a woman get out of 2 minutes of copulation? Most men do not even last that long inside a woman. Such sex leaves the woman dissatisfied and empty, devoid of any form of joy from an otherwise joyful situation.

Lovemaking is not a momentary action. Lovemaking and sexual satisfaction takes hours to build up from the female perspective. The best sexual organ of the body, the brain, prepares you several hours before the actual physical sexual copulation happens. Women want to be talked to or, rather, communicated with sexually long before the actual sex. Women want to be satisfied sexually. They do not want to be treated as objects for the satisfaction of the males as the kama sutra made them out to be. Male sexual satisfaction is necessary but women also want their satisfaction out of the same sex.

Women want to be given their due sexual enjoyment. Sex is a fact of life no doubt about that. Sex and lovemaking is the spice of life. Sex [very good considerate sex] is as natural as walking, sleeping, and breathing. Sex and lovemaking is the lifeblood and the bond that holds together men and women -- marriages and relationships. The ultimate expression of intimacy, sex also is the core of procreation, the way humanity ensures that the human race continues. And for most couples, sex is a source of enjoyment and fellowship. So, why should the womenfolk be denied their enjoyment and fellowship from sex?

Female Kama Sutra - What Today's Woman Wants from Sex

The following are what women want from sex and how they want to be treated before and after sex. When you give your woman what she wants, you are promoting female kama sutra, the sexual satisfaction for women:

•Sex is a seduction of the mind - mental foreplay is crucial to sexual satisfaction for a woman.

•Women want to be romanced and courted always -

women want to know that they are always relevant in your life. Court women with affection and communication.

•Flatter your woman with desire - perceived desire does wonder to the female psyche.

•Women want to be pampered and cherished. Occasional flowers and "i love you" texts or calls or cards are important to women.

•A loving and considerate man who is not afraid to explore the female anatomy and break sexual boundaries to the female multiple orgasms

•A man who is macho enough to help the woman out with perceived female chores.

•A man who knows how to give the females sexual satisfaction always.

•A man who can give head is a darling always.

Give your woman sexual satisfaction today and join in writing the female kama sutra that will be read tomorrow. Do not deny women sexual satisfaction.

THE KAMA SUTRA - NOT JUST A SEX MANUAL

Anyone who has been to India or has read enough about India would have seen ancient Indian sculptures or pictures of them; even someone with the most rudimentary idea about India would we familiar with the Kama Sutra. If you have visited temples like Khajuraho and many others in India, you would have seen frescoes and sculptures featuring exceedingly sexual, even orgiastic postures, various sex positions, even group sex, and same-sex scenes.

In the old days, India faced the problem of underpopulation (as against overpopulation today). So the kings routinely commissioned the court sculptors to design sculptures so erotic that they acted as an aphrodisiac to encourage people to produce more babies to populate their land! Perhaps the Kama Sutra had just such a beginning.

In the west, the Kama Sutra is viewed as an ancient sex manual only, which is it, but it is much more than that. It is also a book about social values, etiquette, duties, economic obligations, etc. Understandably the sex manual part of this voluminous work is what has gained maximum popularity. The Kama, simply put is sex, but more specifically it means enjoyment using all the five senses of touch, taste, smell, hearing and smell and enjoyment not just for the body but for the mind and spirit as well.

One part of the manual deals with sexual positions, how to embrace and kiss, foreplay (marking with nails is one chapter), role-playing and even the appropriate sounds to be made! One entire segment is devoted to advising about how to acquire a wife, another segment is about other people's wives! Another segment is allocated to courtesans, how they should earn money, how to live to behave and conduct themselves, how to live as a man's wife etc.

The final part of the text deals with personal adornment and love potions and other methods of making a person attractive. It also deals with methods of arousal and miscellaneous experiments. All in all, I would conclude that it was a book way ahead of its times.

Some years back a film was made about the period of Indian history when the Kama Sutra was written. It was a film called Utsav and was set in the period of Vatsyayana (the author). This film was about the renowned courtesan of the time, Vasantsena; the haunting melodious songs of the film are still very popular. Courtesans were, in those days viewed with respect, insofar as sex was viewed as an art to be learned and taught. Some parts of the film were very funny too when Vatsayana is shown peering into various rooms of a brothel collecting material for his book.

So really sex was not talked of in hushed tones the way it is now; it was as much part of social life as anything else and the Kama Sutra perhaps best reflects this.

THE SEXUAL (AND NON-SEXUAL) ASPECTS OF THE KAMA SUTRA

The Kama Sutra is an ancient text, originally written in Sanskrit, that has become very closely associated with the sexual aspects of tantra- rightly or wrongly. There are thirty-six chapters in the book, organized into seven parts.

The Introductory Section includes a description of the book's contents, an explanation of the three priorities and aims of life, how to acquire knowledge and the proper conduct for a "well-bred townsman". There are also notes on "intermediaries" that assist the lover go about his tasks.

The second section, On sexual union, is the part of the book that most people are curious about. There are descriptions of desire stimulation and the different types of embraces, caresses, and kisses. There are instructions for the use of fingernails and teeth in sexual activities. Moaning and the positioning of the female body during intercourse are also a topic. Foreplay, behavior during and after coitus are discussed. Sixty-four different sex acts are described in detail.

The third section deals with acquiring a wife. The different types of marriage are discussed. Explanations are given on how to relax, obtain, manage and marry a woman. The following fourth section deals with what to do with that wife when you have her. This includes proper treatment and etiquette.

The fifth section deals with the wives of other people. The behavior of both genders is addressed. Etiquette regarding forums and relationships is discussed in detail. The next section is dedicated to courtesans- more specifically, how to choose, pay and retain your sex worker of choice. The last section describes how to attract others through physical attractiveness and strong sexual confidence.

The text emphasizes what was known as the purusharthas, or the four main goals of life. The first is dharma or the act of living with virtue. The second, Artha, deals with material prosperity. The Kama relates to erotic and aesthetic pleasures. Moksha is liberation through being released from the cycle of life and death. The first three goals can be achieved in everyday life and are ordered according to importance (yes, sex is the least important).

The Kama Sutra is not by definition a tantric text as it does not discuss the sacred rites that are meant to accompany those acts. But many who follow tantra do use the book as a guideline or starting point from which they can build their tantric rituals. The sexuality that is included in this book is meant to correspond to that notion of Kama.

Though it does have a religious nature, the Kama Sutra has been translated into virtually every language on earth. Modified versions of the book exist that only include the sexual aspects often including detailed illustrations or pictures to help the reader achieve what is being described. This sort of textual editing does remove the overall point of the book, which is that sexuality- while rightly one of life's goals- isn't the most important goal and should be handled with consideration to the goals that come before it.

KAMA SUTRA SEX TIPS TO INCREASE PENIS SENSATION

When it comes to masturbation and sex, it is easy to get into a rut. Guys know what feels good and often use the same technique over and over to get the job done. The problem is that going at it the same way every time can eventually lead to overall diminished sexual pleasure and this. in turn, can lead to sexual compensation in the form of frequent masturbation or aggressive sex and both of these sexual activities put stress on penis skin and neurons. The result of this type of sexual behavior is diminished penis sensation.

The best way to solve this problem of sexual redundancy is to mix things up, using positions and techniques that are designed to maximize penis sensation and increase erotic pleasure. Following the ancient secrets of the ama sutra and nourishing the skin of the penis using a mixture of penis-specific vitamins and minerals can increase the receptivity of the erogenous skin and turn the regular bump and grind into a sensual experience to remember.

Why does Penis Sensitivity Diminish Over Time?

The skin of the penis is constantly exposed to friction of one kind or another. Frequent masturbation and sex put a lot of stress on the delicate dermal tissue, and even when men are not active, clothing and other materials can chafe and rub the skin. This ongoing friction causes a toughened layer of skin to build up, like the callouses that develop on the palms of the hands and soles of the feet. Because of this, the nerve endings that underlie the skin of the penis are less able to experience sexual stimuli, leading to decreased pleasure.

To prevent loss of sensitivity or to stimulate new nerve receptors, sex therapists often recommend trying new positions. The Kama Sutra, which is considered by many as the "bible" of sex positions, offers countless new ways to enjoy the erotic play. This unique guide to sexual positions was written over 2,000 years ago, yet men and women have been using these ancient techniques for centuries to enhance the experience of physical pleasure, both during foreplay and intercourse itself.

Introducing the Nirvana

For men who are a little less sensitive down there, this position is ideal and the perfect introduction to the world of the kama sutra. To practice the "Nirvana" position, the woman lies down on a bed and raises her arms over her head - holding on to the headboard is helpful here. Then the man positions himself on top of her. Her thighs remain together, and he straddles her, then enters her in this position. The Nirvana is ideal for both partners, as it not only creates a gentle pressure on the penis but also maximizes the stimulation of the clitoris.

Make the most of the Erotic Experience

In addition to experimenting with new positions such as the one described here, setting the right atmosphere can help both partners to experience sensual pleasure in a new way. Taking time with each other and experimenting with other types of touch beyond penetration can help make the final moment more powerful. Massaging the penis with a specialized vitamin formula for increasing erotic sensation can become a pleasurable part of the experience and can enhance the sensitivity of the penile skin, especially when a partner participates in this sensual moment.

Essential Nutrients For Increased Penis Sensation

A specially designed penis health formula (most health professionals recommend Man1 Man Oil) containing vitamins, minerals, and all-natural moisturizers can be the perfect accompaniment when experimenting with the kama sutra. Vitamins and minerals that improve the tone and texture of the penis skin, such as vitamins A, C, D and B5, along with high-quality moisturizers that improve the skin's natural elasticity and enhance penile sensitivity, can help to increase the receptivity of the nerve cells and take the erotic journey in a whole new direction.

KAMA SUTRA SEX POSITIONS FOR A SMALL PENIS - MAKE HER SATISFIED WITH A SMALL MEMBER

Worry about your performance in bed because you are a small man? Don't fret. With a little tweak and imagination, you too can make the most out of a small member and make her satisfied. Now, if you are not born with the desired endowment, read on as we reveal three stellar small penis positions from the ancient sex bible Kama Sutra.

Wait! Don't enter until you read this...

In the teaching of Kama Sutra, it stressed the importance of foreplay as a way of preparing couples for sex. The foreplay described in Kama Sutra encompasses caressing, touching, kissing, and oral sex. If you don't "warm" her up via long and sensual orgasm, it is very hard for her to climax during sex. Thus, you should never rush foreplay.

Small Penis Sex Positions

•White Tiger

In this position, she arches her back and supports the upper body with forearms. Then, you grasp her buttock and slowly enter from behind. When you thrust, she lowers her chest and keeps her leg close to intensify orgasmic response and supercharge pleasure.

•The Gaping Position

She lies on her back and wraps her legs around your waist. You kneel between her legs and hold her buttock to ensure her pelvis meets the penis. Then, you move your hips back and forth. You may adjust the height of her lower body to ensure great heights for both of you.

•The Elephant Posture

She lies on her stomach, with a big cushion under her body. You lie on top of her body and support yourself with hands. Then, you thrust from the back in slow motion. When you are fully inside her, have her to press her thighs closely.

100% natural. No pills, no device, no surgery reQuired.

THE KAMA SUTRA AND BEYOND - SACRED SEXUALITY TEXTS FROM ANCIENT CULTURES

The Kama Sutra is fairly well known in Western culture but it isn't well known that there are many other erotic books from the past. Well-established cultures, throughout the world, have had an integrated sex-science-spirit connection. Healthy living included a robust sex life that often integrated breathing, movement, ecstatic intimacy techniques, communion with the 'Divine' and lifestyle enhancements that boosted longevity.

From earliest records the Japanese, Chinese, Persians, Arabs, Hindus, Nepalese, Egyptian, South Pacific Islanders and even many Native American tribes had elaborate systems encouraging and promoting high sexual practices. The benefits of good, abundant sex are numerous. These books were manuals on lovemaking and they included guides for couples on kissing, touching, positions in lovemaking, attitudes, moral obligations, and much more. Let's explore a few of these cultures and the 'books' they developed that continue to inform us even today.

•The Kama Sutra

A man named Vatsyayana wrote the Kama Sutra in India, sometime between 200 and 400 AD. It was originally an oral tradition and went through several iterations before being written in the form of 'aphorisms' or short 'sayings' that introduced young men and women to the arts of love and relationship. The original Sanskrit version has been translated many times but its first translator was Sir Richard Burton who was an adventurer and scholar living in Victorian England. He traveled, studied and translated many erotic manuals but today we have very few of his original translations because at his death (1890) his conservative wife burned the remaining translations and original manuscripts he had worked on. Only these few have survived.

•The Perfumed Garden

The Perfumed Garden was written in Arabia in the sixteenth century by Sheikh Nefzawi and translated by Sir Richard Burton. He finished the translation the day before he died. It includes a treatise on the many different sizes and shapes of penises and vaginas (lingam and yoni in Sanskrit). Accordingly, it details thirty-five types of lingams and thirty-eight types of yonis. Written primarily for men, it counsels them to ask the woman for instruction on giving her pleasure. It also contains teaching stories of various sorts, uses humor to get points across and includes many intercourse positions.

•The Ananga Ranga

The Ananga Ranga was written in the sixteenth century in India by a man named Kalyana Malla and first translated by Sir Richard Burton. Whereas the Kama Sutra was written for men and women the Ananga Ranga was written for husbands and not necessarily their wives. The middle-ages, in India, were more repressed and strict and a wife 'belonged' to her husband at this time in history. The Ananga Ranga details ethics and morals, seduction techniques, sexual positions, hygiene, rituals and sexual spells, aphrodisiacs, and other erotic concepts. It pays particular attention to the woman learning to control her pelvic floor muscles to heighten the experience between her husband and her self.

•The Secrets of the Jade Bed Chamber

Many erotic books were written in China during the 28 years of the Sui Dynasty. A return to Taoist practices fueled the prolific writing that included recipes for potency remedies, exotic positions, and counseling in the ways of love. These books included: The Secret Methods of the Plain Girl, Handbook of Sex of the Dark Girl, Recipes of the Plain Girl, Secret Prescriptions for the Bedchamber, Principles of Nurturing and the Secrets of the Jade Chamber. As with many societies that included eroticism in their cultural heritage, there is symbolism in the words selected for use in the books and by lovers. A Jade Stalk meant a man's lingam, whereas a Jade Garden meant the woman's yoni. Taoist practices like ejaculation mastery and breathing exercises were wide-spread and considered health benefits as well as sexual aids.

•The Ishimpo

The Ishimpo was a detailed medical manual that originated in Japan. A portion of it was the erotic teaching manual for that culture as sex and health were intermingled in most Asian cultures. Similar to its counterparts in India and other parts of Asia, it depicted the sex act between man and woman as the essential force that controlled the universe. It expressed the importance of making love as the force in nature that keeps the earth circling the heavens and bodies healthy and vital. Taoism from China was influential to the book and the culture.

•Pillow Books

China, Japan, and most eastern cultures had what is termed "Pillow Books" in addition to the teaching manuals mentioned above. These books were used by couples as erotic stimulants and as reminders of a human's vast sexual potential. The 1001 Arabian Nights tales, translated also by Sir Richard Burton, is one such book. They could be used when a couple got into a rut in their sexual and sensual relating. Pillow Books were adorned with beautiful erotic pictures, poetry, writings, and suggestions that couples could partake of together to stir their passions.

In the last fifteen years, the availability of sexuality on how-to and erotic educational books has become much greater. The interest in expanding sexual knowledge and investigating new, erotically stimulating practices is fueled by DVDs, books, audio programs and a growing body of workshops. Teachers from many different traditions are coming forth to make these teachings available to others. Even as the Baby Boomers have carried the heightened sexual appeal of the 60's forward so the next generations have brought up the energy to investigate and examine anew the benefits and experiences of great sex. With the principles of Mind/Body/Spirit driving the enthusiasm for health, wisdom, and consciousness today, the inclusion of sexuality is being seen as the energy force behind the movement.

THE KAMA SUTRA - GUIDANCE FOR SEX AND MUCH MORE

Many have heard of the Kama Sutra, and if asked, cannot even tell you what it is. Those who answer, often say it's an ancient Indian sex manual, but this is not *q*uite correct.

Indeed the Kama Sutra is from ancient India, and it does contain some description of sexual positions, but the work itself is a life guide for a man; from his childhood till old age.

It considers in one chapter sexual positions, but the other chapters are concerned with those things a man needs to pass through life well.

All too often in our Western society, young men and women learn about their sexuality from other young people, or now films (and books) but these methods often leave the young person perplexed.

Seduction

Seduction usually means where a man (or woman) is guided by their sexual desire and persuades the object of that desire into the sexual union. The seducer is generally thought to be acting out of lust rather than love.

Seduction is practiced by those who possess either power, money, or specialized use of psychological persuasion over another person. In our society, it is full of negative connotations.

In fact, in Western society seduction was, and often still is, frowned upon. In classical India, it was not and indeed considered an art of manliness.

Instructions from the Kama Sutra

Based somehow on the then (and still prevalent thought) that the soul itself is seduced by God Presence (the Krishna epic stories), the man is taught how to seduce and sexually con*q*uer his object of affection.

Not unlike today's scenarios, the man was told to keep a good appearance, perfume himself with costly scents, and present his best image. He was told to create a romantic atmosphere, wherein flowers were present, delicate sweets offered, and potent wines. The advice extended to conversations that were loaded with implications of love and desire. The lighting should be low, and if during the day, a romantic shade should be constructed.

Men should, after plying his prey with the various temptations, seek to slowly make some light, physical contact. This can extend to the simple touching of a hand or arm, to more. If a kiss were possible, to kiss.

Seduction and Not Foreplay

Whereas foreplay is a constituent part of the sexual act, seduction here stops with physical contact. Seduction is meant to create a desire where there was none before. Seduction is meant to kindle the fire of passion.

There is a very thin line drawn in Western thought, between a seducer and a rapist. In ancient India, rape would have been considered an unforgivable sin, and often punished with death. Seduction, on the other hand, was an art form, and being so (and still being so) was practiced by masters. Indeed there are two meanings. In the Kama Sutra, seduction means an act of winning the love or sexual favor of someone.

KAMA SUTRA KISSING TECHNIQUES - KNOW THE SECRETS

They are some great Kama Sutra Techniques you can use with kissing and foreplay that will help your partner have a mind-blowing orgasm. It is important to know that using kissing before sex can intensify the orgasm a woman will have because it gets her in the mood quicker. Also, a woman has several areas of her body that are very sensitive to kissing and using these techniques will have your partner begging for more.

A woman's neck is a great place to start when you are wanting to get her in the mood quickly. You can kiss her gently on her neck and this will make her stimulated. It is important to take your time and enjoy what you are doing and most importantly do not rush it, this will only get her out of the mood and will not make for a great lovemaking experience.

You want to use your tongue as well when kissing her because it is warm and stimulating to the touch. The side of her neck and then down her back is a place to get her stimulated. You should also take advantage of kissing her in her thigh area because this will get her lower area warmed up before sex.

Your gentle kiss if done correctly can give her an orgasm even before sex. It is always important to know the secrets of kissing and what makes a woman have an orgasm. You should get all the information you can so that you will have the best experience that you can when trying new things.

EASY KAMA SUTRA - FOR THE BEGINNERS

If you are new to lovemaking, these easy Kama Sutra positions will be ideal for you to try out with your partner. These positions that we are going to discuss will require minimum effort from both partners while getting the most pleasure out of it.

•The Scissor Position

The woman will lie down with her back on the bed, while the man will kneel in front of her. He will then hold her legs wide at the ankles and penetrate her from his kneeling position. This position allows deep penetration which makes it highly stimulating for the man. Do place a cushion underneath the woman's hips to make her feel more comfortable.

•The Tonkin Delight Position

The woman lies on her back, bending her knees and her legs open. The man will slide in between her legs and lift her hips slightly for easier penetration. This position is ideal for the man to easily reach over to her abdomen to caress and kiss it, while the woman just lies back and enjoys.

•The Scandinavian Position

The man will lie down and the woman will kneel astride her partner, with her back facing him. He will then hold her waist and thrusts, while she slides up and down on him. In this position, the woman's hands are free to play with his scrotum, while the man is free to caress her buttock.

*The Beat Position

This is a variation to the legendary missionary position. The woman lies with her legs wide open and the man will place a cushion underneath her hips to tilt the vagina for deeper penetration. Then, the man will go on top of her and penetrate her. He will use his hands to take off his weight and control the thrusting movement as well. This position is highly intimate and stimulating for both partners, allowing the couple to embrace and caress each other.

To enjoy making love, you will not always need to execute complicated sexual positions. Sometimes, easy positions such as those mentioned above can also be pleasurable and stimulating for you and your partner.

WHAT IS THE PSYCHOLOGY BEHIND THE KAMA SUTRA?

The Kama Sutra is an ancient text written by Vatsyayana around the 2nd CAD in India. He was of the Vedic tradition, from which the Trinity god made its way into Christianity. Before writing and printing, there were images in stone that show exotic sexual poses, such as in the Hindi sex temples at Khajuraho. While they show an obsession with sexual pleasure the reason behind them is the psychology born of a desire to fertilize the Mother God.

This is now such a way-out proposition that many would dismiss it as fanciful. The facts, however, speak of a time when men were so obsessed with their fertilizing abilities that they dreamed big and the modern faiths are born of them. The one mystery that all men have dealt with throughout history has been that of sex.

It was not only a *q*uestion of what drives it but of the physical changes in a man's body when passion and desire take charge of it. The penis became the most used symbol in ancient societies and all over Europe the 'menhirs' stand as a testimony. Some are positioned in such a way that the sun forms a star on the peak of it.

Mountains are considered places of holiness because here when the sun passes behind the peak it forms a star. The seven-point and five-point stars are designed on this image and they remain a symbol of Mother God.

The psychology of men able to use their male organs in this way was the purpose of contests. 'Semen' is derived from 'see-man' and one can only imagine the types of challenges that were invented to show how much of the magic fluid one could produce, and how often. The winner was the 'hero' or 'her circle'. In other words, he passed through the circle to 'marry' Mary and live as her consort from then on.

Mary was the name of the Mother-god in Babylon and here, as in other cities, walls of breasts were displayed to caress and introduce fore-play into the marriage. The images in the Kama Sutra and the temples of India, Japan, and elsewhere, are reminders that this is what lies behind the philosophy of religions.

My reincarnation demonstrates that there are no such places as heaven and hell but that they are weapons to force people to accept the beliefs of our ancestors. The psychology is still based on reconciliation with the god in heaven and to make men powerful. It also has the effect of turning women into chattels and forcing them to cover up. That way their presence is less offensive to the sun.

As verification of how influential the sun is in religions, the old symbolism and associated names tell the story. In ancient rock art, such as found in the Nordic Countries, men are depicted rising upwards with a cross either on their bodies or as a kite lifting them. This symbol is encircled to display both symbols as related to crucifixion. Those who supposedly passed on in this way were drawn with them above their heads.

They are then terms 'san't' for 'sun's cross' and this became 'saint'. 'San' stands for sun, saint, and son, in many languages as a remnant of its origin. Sanskrit, the original language of Hindi, is from 'san-script' or 'sun written' and its early form is with signs taken from the sun. These are made as shadows, stars, and so on.

Men dying on crosses also made signs and sounds that found their way into language through interpretation by a high priest or Sharman. He was considered to be in close relationship with the sun and, therefore, able to pass on her messages. It is also the reason why 'holy men' in India are usually found on the peaks where they remain in close connection with the celestial body.

Their role is one of psychologically enforcing the will of the Mother God over those who seek help or knowledge. For this reason, they are kept by the community which supplies them with food and other essentials for their life and comfort.

ASIAN EROTIC MASSAGE - HOW TO EXPERIENCE KAMA SUTRA PLEASURE AND A TASTE OF THE EXOTIC

Getting a massage is a wonderful experience. It helps to calm you and relax you and it can be the perfect end to a troubling day. There is a vast array of massages out there, and few are as good as the Asian erotic massage. The Asian erotic massage is the perfect type of massage for you and your partner because it allows you both to find your erogenous zones while using the principles of tantric massage and the legendary Kama Sutra.

The main principle of the Asian erotic massage is finding the zones of the body that provide pleasure. Now, it is important to point out that when we talk about an Asian erotic massage, we are not talking about illegal massage parlors that can be found in most cities. This is a massage that does not have sex included in it, but it will help you relax like no other massage can.

There are a vast number of books that have been printed on the concept of the Asian erotic massage and the history of the massage dates back thousands of years to China, where it was often used as holistic medicine practice. The body was thought to have a life force by the Chinese and Southeast Asians, and one way to work with that life force was to touch the areas of the body where the force was the strongest. Not surprisingly, those areas were also highly sexual areas and the Asian erotic massage was born.

The Asian erotic massage is much like a tantric massage in that it helps to put you in an incredibly relaxing trance. Many people find they seem to drift not into sleep, but into a waking sleep where they feel what is going on but are reaching almost another level of consciousness. This was also how the Kama Sutra worked, allowing people to reach sexual ecstasy while at the same time expanding their minds and their spirits.

As with so many things in East Asia, the Asian erotic massage is more than just a massage. It is a spiritual experience that helps to align the Chi and helps to make you feel as though you are moving to another plane of existence. With this massage, you can become closer to your partner on a deeper level than you ever thought possible. It is a massage that is more than a massage. It is a trance-like experience that you have to experience to truly believe.

ORAL SEX - THE KAMA SUTRA WAYS

The best way to keep a woman is to continuously shower her with unforgettable sex. To become a great lover, you must master the stimulation techniques via oral sex. When done properly, it can lead her to mind-boggling orgasm. It's no wonder why some women prefer oral sex to lovemaking. In this article, we will discuss a few oral sex tips from the ancient Indian text, Kama Sutra.

*Mr. Clean

According to Kama Sutra, cleanliness should be the number one priority for all lovers. To make her feel comfortable with you, you need to look good, smell nice and taste nice. Before a long and hot oral session, take a warm shower. Don't forget to trim your fingernails as you don't want to cause discomfort to her tender body.

*Setting the Mood

According to experts, it takes 20 minutes of arousal time before a woman can orgasm. Thus, you need to start slow. Kiss and touch her all over the body before you make your move to the genital.

*Teasing Technique

It's a powerful technique to turn her on. Here's how it works: kiss and lick her inner thigh gently. Meanwhile, use your fingers to stroke the area around the genital. Hold off from coming in contact with her genital until she requests you to do so.

*Clitoral Stimulation

Using the rip of your tongue, stroke her perineum in a circular motion. As she is getting more excited, lick and suck the clitoris gently. Be very gentle as the clitoris is the most sensitive area of women.

COMBINE EXERCISE, STRETCHING AND KAMA SUTRA AND YOU GET EXERSUTRA

My wife and I were making love one night, nothing was feeling good, it was stale, boring, average and just so routine. After we rushed through it and cleaned up, I asked her how I was performing. Well, she loved that I used my hands and tongue to caress her body but other than that I was a failure. She then asked me what I felt about her performance. I was a bit mad from what she said so I just blasted out "Well to be honest it's getting boring!"

After a three-day fight, lousy make-up sex, and then a 3-hour talk we both decided to change our lifestyle so we can improve not only our sex life but our relationship as well. Let's face it, sex brings us closer together with our significant other. You bond intimately and emotionally. A healthy sex life also leads to more confidence and less stress when handling your day-to-day business. When I have a great lovemaking session I tend to wake up the next day refreshed, focused and ready to take on the day.

So what plan was put into motion to save our relationship and bring back the passion? Well for starters we stopped eating fast food, restaurants and stopped drinking soda cold turkey. We started going to the gym every night. We even started having sex every night. Sure we were losing weight, getting healthier and had more energy for sex, but sex was still the same as before. What were we doing wrong?

Well after another two months of trying to improve our sex life I stopped mid-sex one night and told her to stop. My right leg was cramping and all I could think about was the pain in my leg! It was killing my motivation and focus and I was having a hard time keeping a solid erection. She admitted that me not being fully hard was also making her think that I was not into her and that was all she could think about.

My wife knows I love her and I know she loves me. We were getting in better shape and we were rediscovering our sexual attraction for each other but that wasn't the issue. I told her that I think we need to try more positions until we find one that works for both of us. We must have gone through ten different kama sutra books before we gave up. These positions were hard! I was not a professional porn start and neither was she. How can they have an orgasm when it feels like you are working out, not having sex?!

Finally one day I was searching the internet for sexual exercising and I came across this poorly designed website called ExerSutra. I thought you know what, I am going to give this a shot. The webpage talked about combining exercising, stretching and balance into your sexual positions. This made sense to me because even though we were jogging every day at the gym and building more endurance, we were still cramping and having sex was uncomfortable and we couldn't stay in the same position for more than two minutes without having to switch.

ExerSutra was a cheap guide that combined exercising methods to achieve more endurance for the advanced sexual positions with stretching techniques so you are not cramping up. I have to say I was blown away and my eyes were opened! I was so excited that I called in sick to work the next day just to read this guide. I was practicing stretching all day and when my wife got home, I attacked her with my new-found knowledge. I threw her on the bed and went to town. I couldn't believe how long I was lasting. No cramps. No balance issues. She was also loving it, just laying there getting pleasured. For the first time in 8 months, we shared a mutual orgasm.

She asked me where that came from, and I showed her ExerSutra. We immediately changed up our workout routines to include more strength training that targeted the muscle groups more commonly used during intercourse. We stretched before and after our work out and also before and after sex! The night she pulled off a reverse cowgirl and we went for 18 minutes straight in one position was the night I laid in bed with the biggest smirk on my face. I was a man.

KAMA SUTRA - WHAT TO DO AFTER READING KAMA SUTRA?

Kama Sutra is one book which records all the various sexual positions that one can try out with his or her partner. In Kama Sutra, some positions are not commonly practiced by couples. Couples are not sure what they are missing out on as these Kama Sutra positions will give them a new sense of fulfillment and excitements when practiced.

You may be thinking that after you have read the Kama Sutra manual, you will be able to be a sex expert on the bed. This is usually not the truth. The Kama Sutra manual can only illustrate with the help of pictures, tell you what are the possible techniques and positions that you can try out with your partner.

To have a more than satisfaction and passionate sex, you will need to understand more about sexuality way beyond the Kama Sutra manual. There are other important elements that you cannot miss out on if you want to create the perfect sex experience with your partner.

One of them is passion. Passion is an intangible thing, it is a feeling. By using good sexual positions and techniques in the bedroom does not guarantee that your sexual ride will be passionate enough. But with creative and erotic ideas, you will be able to apply it in your bedroom, and thus making the whole sexual experience to be more fun and fresh.

So what to do after reading Kama Sutra manual? Spend some time to get more ideas to increase the passion and intimacy with your lover. Combine those ideas with the

Kama Sutra positions that you have learned in the manual, and you will be able to surprise and delight your lover.

CONCLUSION

Any time you desire some aid boosting your sex life, the Kama Sutra handbook can support you! The areas in the Kama Sutra are incredibly attention-grabbing regarding men and women requiring a little help inside the bedroom or throughout their relationship. Even if you're not experiencing problems within your present sex life or relationship this handbook can be hugely beneficial, even if you just make use of it, to begin with for the sexual positions. Wanting to improve your partnership by making use of techniques from the Kama Sutra is entirely normal. Learn the Kama Sutra with your lover, you will certainly discover this very helpful as you can agree or even disagree with some enhancements in which require to be made inside your romance.

Mood setting is very beneficial, it aids you to see deep into your lover as well as feel exactly how they are feeling. Closeness together with your partner is mostly produced simply by setting the mood. Trying to keep things easy in a mood-setting is fantastic! A good bit of music as well as sweet-talking your lover is the ideal mood setting. One of the most well-known ways is to light some fragrant candles or plain candles and incense sticks or burners. Best of all this is cost-effective. You can pick these types of things up for very little these days and are common. Make sure the particular area your planning to use is smelling clean and looking excellent is an additional fantastic approach.

Good smelling bedding is a key element, no one wants stinky bed sheets while trying to make love. Feeling calm and comfortable is key, so having the room is fresh and thoroughly clean is a must.

9 781712 903889